C000115432

WALKING BACK TO
HAPPINESS

THE SECRET TO ALCOHOL-FREE LIVING & WELL-BEING

NIGEL JONES

First published in Great Britain in 2022
9KM BY 9AM Publishing
The Purple Tangerine Limited
82 The High Street
Charing
Kent
United Kingdom
TN27 0LS
www.9kmby9am.com/books

© Copyright Nigel Jones, 2022

The moral right of the author has been asserted.

All rights reserved. Without limiting the rights under copyright reserved above, no part of this publication may be reproduced, stored or introduced into a retrieval system, or transmitted, in any form or by any means (electronic, mechanical, photocopying, recording or otherwise), without the prior written permission of both the copyright owner and the publisher of this book.

A CIP catalogue of this book is available from the British Library.

ISBN 978-1-915147-30-1 – Paperback
ISBN 978-1-915147-31-8 – Hardback
eISBN 978-1-915147-32-5 – Ebook

First Edition

This book is the personal experience of the author. It is not intended as a substitute for professional assistance but describes the author's journey as well as learnings from that journey on stopping the consumption of alcohol for one year and beyond. While the author has used reasonable endeavours to ensure the information contained in the book is accurate and as up to date as possible at the time of publication, medical and well-being knowledge is constantly changing. It is therefore recommended that readers consult a qualified medical and / or professional specialist for individual advice. This book should not be used as an alternative to seeking medical or other professional advice concerning alcohol, habits, addiction or any of the topics covered herein, which should be sought before any action is taken as a result of reading this book. The author and publisher cannot be held responsible for any actions that may be taken by a reader as a result of any reliance on the information contained in the book, which is taken entirely at the reader's own risk.

DEDICATION

To my mum, Lucy, a true Stoic and the strongest,
most determined person I know.

To my wife, Heather, and children, Liberty,
Verity and Leo. You are my world.

To my father-in-law, Michael Stewart,
for your wise words and attention to detail.

Thank you Ruari and Andy for giving me the
opportunity to get my life back.
I will be forever grateful.

Jaynie Bye – the best Editor in the world
Heather Stewart-Jones – Illustrations
Anthony Pike – Design

SPECIAL THANKS

To all the people (living and deceased) who were an influence on me in writing this book including: Roy Baumeister, Craig Beck, Holly J. Bertone, Stephan Bodian, Tara Brach, Russell Brand, Arthur C. Brooks, Gudrun Buhnemann, Joseph Campbell, James Clear, Pema Chödrön, Jack Kornfield, The Dalai Lama, Charles Duhigg, Tim Ferriss, Rabbi Finley, Dan Harris, Henry Ford, Viktor Frankl, Robert Frost, Julia Galef, Chris Gardner, Annie Grace, Rick Hanson, William Ernest Henley, Ryan Holiday, Arianna Huffington, Gary Keller, Beth Kempton, Jonathan Landaw, Dr. Qing Li, Catarino Lino, Abraham Maslow, Matthew McConaughey, Kelly McGonigal, Dan Millman, Walter Mischel, Carl Newport, Ivan Pavlov, Rafael Pelayo, Anthony Robbins, Rich Roll, John Seabrook, Martin Seligman, Dan Siegel, Baba Shiv, Pedram Shojai, Henry David Thoreau, Eckhart Tolle, Bronnie Ware, Alan Watts and Chris Wilson.

CONTENTS

INTRODUCTION

'Under the floor of some poor man's house lies a treasure. But because he does not know of its existence, he does not think he is rich. Similarly, inside one's mind lies truth itself, firm and unfading. Yet because beings see it not, they experience a constant stream of misery. The treasure of truth lies within the house of the mind.'

Buddhist Teaching

'As a single footstep will not make a path on the earth, so a single thought will not make a pathway in the mind. To make a deep physical path, we walk again and again. To make a deep mental path, we must think over and over the kind of thoughts we wish to dominate our lives.'

Henry David Thoreau

PREFACE

MY STORY

This is the story of how a 50-something-year-old, who had been locked into the habit of drinking alcohol for over 35 years, finally woke up and said, 'I want a different life'; how he found his purpose and in doing so, transformed his mind and body; how he lost 30% of his body weight and made anxiety and sleepless nights a thing of the past.

Set out over six sections, the book follows my experiences over the first year of alcohol-free living, covering:

- Time To Act: Day One
- The Journey Begins: The First Few Days
- Discovering The New You: The First Few Weeks
- Understanding The New You: The First Few Months
- The New You: Beyond 90 Days
- A New Life: One Year & Beyond

Each chapter comprises...

- My Story
- What I Learnt
- Steps You Can Take
- Key Learnings

On a Monday evening, early in December, I had my final drink. I did not know it was my final one at the time, but lying in bed the next morning I signed up to the One Year No Beer (OYNB) 28-Day Challenge to stop drinking all alcohol (not just beer). There were also 90-Day and 365-Day Challenges, but on that Tuesday morning, I committed to 28 days. I was going to do it.

One of the amazing, unbelievable changes that happened to me almost immediately after quitting, was that I started to feel alive and much, much happier than I had done for years. I had so much energy. I was waking up at around five o'clock, full to the brim with 'get up and go'.

Six months down the line, this energy had translated itself into walking at least nine kilometres every day before 9 o'clock. I called this 9KM BY 9AM.

Following a 9KM BY 9AM lifestyle is like putting a scaffolding structure around the house that is my body and mind. It provides me with the opportunity to live both a physically and mentally fit life, and allows me to build, repair and refurbish 'my house'.

9KM BY 9AM is how I challenge myself. It has become the way I live my life. At its heart, it is about doing something challenging early in the day. For me, it is walking 9km. For others, it could be walking 1km, running 2km, cycling 10km, writing a song, reading a book, painting a landscape – everyone is different.

Every day, I now get up and do some work on 'my house'!

WHAT I LEARNT

To me, stopping drinking alcohol is akin to going on an adventure – a hero's adventure.

This book is about my journey, my adventure, to a new life of alcohol-free living.

It's a story many can relate to, irrespective of age or gender. Whether male or female, in your 20s, 30s, 40s, 50s, 60s, 70s or even 80s, it's never too late to go on this alcohol-free journey.

STEPS YOU CAN TAKE

By choosing an alcohol-free life, you change your story.

My story is about the obstacles I have faced and the wisdom I gained. I do hope it helps you on your path to this new and wonderfully rich life that alcohol takes away from so many.

This book is about how I stepped up and now live an alcohol-free life. I hope you will join me by taking your own alcohol-free adventure.

KEY LEARNINGS

This book will help you:

- Identify your values
- Cement your beliefs
- Find your purpose
- Reduce your anxiety
- Lose weight
- Improve your well-being
- Discover the power of mindfulness and meditation
- Be more present
- Unleash your alcohol-free super power
- Transform your body and mind

Nigel Jones

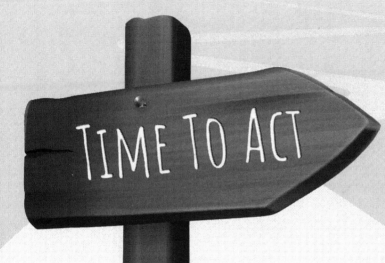

DAY 1

TIME TO ACT: DAY 1

There was something majorly wrong with my life. I was in my mid-50s, and I knew that if I continued along the trajectory I was on, I would be lucky to see my 60th birthday. I was locked in my own *Groundhog Day* existence. I finally admitted to myself that the one thing that was causing all my pain and suffering was the one thing I'd thought for years was helping me: my good friend alcohol.

You don't have to be an alcoholic to stop drinking. You just need to recognise that your relationship with alcohol can lead to life-changing issues – not just for you but for your loved ones, your work colleagues, in fact, everyone you are connected to.

CHAPTER 1
ALCOHOL & ME

Let's make one thing very clear from the start. I was not pouring Whisky on my Weetabix, Malibu on my Muesli or Frascati on my Frosties! I was not drinking out of a brown paper bag. I had, however, weaved alcohol into my life. I was drinking every day. At the end of the relationship, it was the equivalent of around a bottle of wine a day, more on weekends. But still enough to make me feel like there must be more to life.

MY STORY

I have given much thought to the questions: why did I start drinking and why did I continue to drink on a regular daily basis for over 35 years?

I did not consider myself to have a drink problem. Everyone I knew drank. It was the normal thing to do. Friends, work colleagues, relatives, girlfriends, teachers, lecturers, even priests. I could go on.

How much you drink is NOT relevant to anybody else, only you, because it's all about you.

For example, two glasses a night could be highly dangerous to one person and to another it could just be their starter. Everybody is different.

When I stopped drinking, I noticed that the first thing other drinkers ask (or think) is, 'Do you have a problem?'

This is only to make them feel better about themselves. They are just trying to gauge themselves against you.

By stopping drinking, you are a shining beacon. You are doing things differently, taking the path less travelled, wanting a better life. You have decided to leave the tribe. This tends to make anyone staying in the tribe feel uncomfortable. They want to believe the only reason you have stopped is because you have a problem or you have found a new religion! Other drinkers need to put you in a box, label you, and then forget about it. They don't need to ask any more questions. They can go on drinking as normal.

Even with my regular alcohol intake, I ran my own successful marketing agency, have been married for 25 years and have three wonderful, grown-up children. But every day, I was putting this poison inside myself, thinking it was some form of relaxant, stress reliever, anxiety killer.

But I was overweight (well over 17 stone), short of breath, anxious, short-tempered and doing very little exercise. These were all symptoms of too much alcohol consumption and an unhealthy lifestyle.

I did do some exercise but not enough to make an impact on my weight and mental well-being. I went cycling and played golf, always spending time at the 19th hole.

Being in my 50s, my body was not what it used to be. Even two drinks the night before would lead to a hangover. I never really looked at it as a problem until well into my 40s, when my body started to tell me that it just could not cope as it used to with the mental and physical effects.

GROWING UP IN THE 1970s & EARLY 1980s

I don't think much has changed in 50 years regarding the way alcohol is promoted though media.

Even though the amount of information we receive has massively increased in volume through social media, the internet and smartphones, alcohol is still pretty much positioned the same.

When I was a boy, there were only a handful of TV channels – BBC1, BBC2, ITV and, in the early 80s, along came Channel 4. There were national newspapers and local papers, plus magazines. There was also radio – with only a few stations to choose from, including national BBC stations and local independent radio. To watch a movie, you had to go to the cinema. There was no internet.

The home I grew up in was alcohol-free. My mother and father were not drinkers. There was never alcohol in the home apart from at Christmas time when it would appear for a week or so in the form of cans of beer, a bottle of whisky, maybe Malibu and Baileys or a bottle of Advocaat that would become a Snowball if you added lemonade to it! There was no wine. Wine in the UK in the 70s and 80s mainly consisted of a German sweet white wine called Liebfraumilch.

My parents did not drink during the week. On a Saturday night, when they would go out dancing at a local club, it was only a couple of pints of beer. Other than that, I think my dad would have a couple of pints during the week if he went out to play skittles so, in total, he was drinking maybe four pints of beer a week maximum and my mother much less than that. So, my parental role models drank, but hardly anything at all. My older brother, who was 14 years older than me and lived at home until he was 21, did venture to the pub more often, so this probably had some influence on me as a young boy.

Alcohol was very much associated with successful people. Of course, there were the drunk tramps drinking out of bottles concealed in brown paper bags, but they were classed as alcoholics. The very clear message through TV, cinema and all media was that the more successful, rich and famous you were, the more alcohol you could afford. Success was a bar in your house; success was drinking champagne. In sport, it was James Hunt covered in champagne after winning F1; George Best pouring champagne into a pyramid of glasses. In the movies, it was James Bond drinking his Vodka Martini. On TV, it was Leonard Rossiter enjoying a Cinzano Bianco with Joan Collins. Anyone who was successful usually had a drink in their hand.

The TV adverts were creative and appealed to younger people with their catchy slogans, staying sharp to the bottom of the glass, probably the best lager in the world, refreshing the parts other beers cannot reach, follow the bear and reassuringly expensive.

This definitely had an effect on my subconscious mind. I was being groomed. Every media channel was telling me alcohol was good for me. Successful people consumed it. Adults consumed it. It was fun. It made you sociable. You became a fun person if you drank it!

My recollection is that I never thought of drinking alcohol until I was probably around 14 years old.

Outside school, social life consisted of a weekly youth club and the odd disco in a village hall. There weren't many of these, probably four or five a year.

There was definitely pressure among my friends to drink a couple of cans of beer or cider before going to these village hall discos. It was good to have an older and/or taller friend who could get served in an off-licence. We all knew the three or four shops that would sell us cigarettes and beer.

Once the cans of beer were acquired from the shop, they were normally consumed in secret, in a park, somewhere where no one could see. This drinking gave me a slight 'high' and normally ended in me being sick. Nothing like it was portrayed on TV!

In the summer evenings, my parents would take my younger sister and me, not that often but maybe two or three times each year, to pubs with an area for children to play. My father would probably have a couple of drinks, my mother too. My sister and I would play on the swings and slides and have crisps and soft drinks. So, I began to associate pubs with having fun.

On the flip side, I had aunties and uncles who drank a lot. It was not talked about much in the family but word slipped down the grapevine to me that several had 'issues'. My father's older brother was one of these. He still lived with his mother and father well into his 50s. He was a big man, with a full, red face, who was always down the pub. One of my mother's sisters drank a lot of wine. She lived alone and my mother would take me along to visit her on the occasional Saturday morning. Her house was full of empty wine bottles. So I saw first-hand the destruction alcohol causes.

By my teenage years, I was starting to build a belief that alcohol was cool, that drinking it was a normal thing to do. Everybody did it. It was a rite of passage. Grown-ups drank. Everyone else drank, well, most people. It was everywhere. It was hard to avoid. If you did not drink it would be unusual. Suspect. Wrong.

MY FIRST DRINK

The effects were like nothing I'd ever known before. I felt absolutely terrible. The headache was excruciating but it was the start of a long-term relationship that lasted almost 40 years – what a first date!

I was 14 and with my friend, who would've been 16 at the time and lived just around the corner. He had acquired some home-made scrumpy and his parents were out. He invited me round and I drank about two or three pints of the stuff, which was poured out of a plastic carton that looked like a petrol bottle, which is ironic as alcohol is pretty similar to fuel.

I remember the room spinning and me saying that I had to leave. I really thought I was going to die. I staggered home and I think I tried to creep into the house, because I was in such a bad way, but ended up throwing up all over the upstairs hallway. The next day, I had a very bad headache, like nothing I'd ever had before. This was my first hangover.

I would go on to have thousands of these over the following years.

This first drink experience was an end in itself. The only reason we were drinking was to get drunk but I had no idea I was going to get drunk. It was only my older friend who knew what was going to happen. He'd probably been through something similar a few years earlier. It was my rite of passage – I had to do it. Everybody did it.

My second date with alcohol was linked to a village disco. I was still aged only 14. I remember buying four cans of beer and then going to the park to drink them with other friends going to the disco. We knew the places that would sell alcohol to 14-year-olds. I went into the shop, very nervously, with our money and bought the cans of beer. We sat behind some bushes, out of sight so no one could see us drinking. Again, the whole objective was to get drunk and feel high.

Drinking the first few times was, for me, just beer. My first experience with spirits was at a friend's house party. I remember drinking whisky, which tasted disgusting. The hangover was so bad. Throughout the rest of my teens and 20s, I could not drink whisky again as the mere smell of it took me back to that party as a 14-year-old.

Looking back on this, I really should have realised then that it was not the whisky that tasted disgusting – it was the alcohol, the same chemical, or active ingredient, in beer that I had decided I liked.

The only other spirits I drank as a teenager were mixed with a sweet drink like Coca-Cola and the only objective of drinking spirits was to get drunk quicker. But the drink of choice as a teenager became beer.

By 16, drinking was something we always did if we went to a party. I remember being at a holiday camp in Somerset and buying scrumpy from a garage and ending up behind a hedge completely drunk and sick again. Why the hell did I do this? It was just crazy. In fact, most drinking experiences as a teenager ended up with me back in bed by myself with the room spinning around!

By the time I was in the sixth form, there were at least two 18th birthday parties each month at night clubs in the town centre. There were always tickets available, so even if you did not know the person, you would go along to the party where alcohol was readily available and being sold knowingly to 16 and 17-year-olds.

With alcohol all around me, it started to become a regular thing for me when I was about 17. Not that I was drinking it daily but if there was a party, I would almost certainly have a drink. The first thing I did after finishing my A-level exams was to go to the pub to celebrate with other students.

HAPPY HOURS

The second phase of drinking started for me at the age of 18 and coincided with leaving home and going to university. Drinking became an everyday thing.

I've only realised now, while writing this chapter, the power of the Happy Hour slogan. It works on a number of levels. The first level being that you feel happy because drinks are discounted for an hour, so you are saving money and getting more for your hard-earned cash. However, the subliminal message is that alcohol makes you happy. As you will see later in this book, that is a complete load of nonsense.

I went to the London School of Economics and, as with all universities, alcohol was all around me. It was everywhere: Fresher's Week, Happy Hours, Club Welcome Drinks. Everyday drinking became the norm. Weekends were the worst, staying up into the early hours of Saturday morning, sleeping all day Saturday and doing it again Saturday night. For the first term, roughly ten weeks, I drank almost every day. I was not alone. Most people did.

University was the time of my life when the habit was etched into my brain. The only day I did not drink was

Monday, maybe Tuesday, but by Wednesday it was the start of the weekend. It was usually two or three pints of beer during the week and more at the weekend. It was not as if I had the money to do this either. But, somehow, I found a way to fund the drinking, normally through Happy Hours and cheap supermarket wine. I recall a brand called Thunderbird that was 15% ABV. One bottle of this before going out to the student union became the norm.

PROFESSIONAL LIFE

After university, I initially had several short-term jobs before landing what I would call a 'career path' position in one of the top accountancy firms. I stayed for just a year as it was just not the right fit for me. I then went into journalism for around 18 months, finally ending up in one of the world's biggest marketing, advertising and public relations agencies. I stayed in this sector for the next 35 years.

PR had a huge client entertainment side to it. I was effectively being paid to drink with my clients and members of the media.

We worked hard but we also played hard. Client entertainment always involved booze, at long lunches, dinners, parties and meetings. Staying away in hotels meant ending up in the bar until the early hours, and it was all effectively free, that is, I did not pay for it. I even had beer and spirit clients so access to supplies was the norm.

I used to think that it was just the industry I was in that had alcohol playing a central role, but as I listened to others, it became apparent that this legal, addictive drug is a problem in almost all industries. There are the obvious ones like the City, insurance, accountancy, legal and marketing, where client entertaining is paramount, but it has also weaved its way into many business and trade cultures, including the medical profession, teaching, and the police, to name just a few. I am sure that if you look at the industry you work in, alcohol will play a role.

By the time I hit my mid-30s, I had developed a palate for fine wine and was drinking around a bottle of wine a day, maybe one and a half or two a day on weekends. I did not consider myself to have a problem as my colleagues and friends were doing the same.

THE BAR IN THE CELLAR

By my late 30s, I achieved the dream of building a real bar in my own home – in the cellar. It had its own name, a website and a drinks menu. It was like a church of booze, the bar being the altar. It was a statement that I was successful. I'd made it. It was fully stocked with wine, beer and even spirits hanging on the wall behind the bar so you could pour yourself a large one whenever you liked. It was like being in a movie.

The bar was a novelty, a folly. We celebrated my 40th birthday down there. It could hold, at a squeeze, up to 30 people.

I tended to be the barman, pouring everyone's drinks. I really enjoyed it. It was hard work. Non-stop for five or six hours.

By this time, I was running my own company based in an annexe of our main house and the bar was somewhere I could take clients after a meeting for a glass of something. This was to me, at the time, a dream come true. Who was I kidding?

To stock the bar, it cost well over £500 and, at Christmas, maybe even £1,000. I had two of every spirit just in case I ran out and I needed to be able to make any cocktail I was asked for by my guests. There was a house white and red, normally a Chablis and a Cabernet Sauvignon plus a selection of other wines. Stock was always around a minimum of 30 bottles. On top of this, there was a wide selection of beers and soft drinks.

Our three children loved it as they had a lot of their birthday parties there. The bar was given a soft drink overhaul for around three hours and then the adults were invited to pop in for a drink when they picked their children up.

The novelty wore off after a year or so and the bar was only used for Easter, Christmas and the occasional birthday.

The village had one pub so my drinking was pretty much wine at home and two pints down at the local. I probably went to the pub two or three times a week by myself but would meet locals there at the bar.

So, all in all, I was not drinking a massive amount but looking back on it now, it was still a lot.

ABSTINENCE

In the 36 years that I drank alcohol, the longest I went without drinking was six days. I think I did five days three times and a handful of three days. On top of this, there were around 10 alcohol-free days a year. This adds up to around 360 days of non-drinking during my drinking years.

So, in 13,000 days, I didn't drink for 360 days. Of the 360 days I didn't drink, these were probably because I was hungover from the day before when I had drunk twice as much as I should have. Over the 36 years, I drank about 1,000 litres of neat alcohol. Really, I should be dead. In a way, I was dead.

THE LAST DAYS BEFORE THE LAST DAY ONE

By the age of 54, I knew this really had to stop. I knew that what I was doing was crazy. I wanted to stop. I had wanted to stop for about ten years. But now I really wanted to stop. My body was getting older and it just could not take the side effects of alcohol.

Towards the end of my drinking days, I was drinking roughly a half bottle of spirits, seven bottles of wine and six pints of beer each week. My neat alcohol intake per week was 140ml from spirits, 656ml from wine and 199ml from beer. Total 995ml. That's 52 litres a year. I had to stop.

This cycle of behaviour was starting to wear me down. I knew I had to do something but I really did not know how to break free. Something had to change and it did.

WHAT I LEARNT

Putting pen to paper and writing my alcohol life story was an enlightening experience. This story of my relationship with alcohol revealed three main things:

The difficulty of getting hooked. You really have to work hard at it. I remember others saying to me at the start of my drinking career, 'You should try Guinness, it's an acquired taste. You won't like it initially but it will grow on you.' What a load of codswallop.

Are there any other things in my life that I have taken up for over 35 years that initially tasted disgusting and made me sick? The only one I can think of is alcohol.

What seems to be going on here is some form of gigantic conspiracy. Alcohol has weaved its way into almost every aspect of our lives, from celebrating births and marriages, to raising a glass to the lives of those we have lost. If we're happy, we'll drink to celebrate. If we're sad, we'll drink to commiserate. If we're angry, we'll drink to calm down. If we're calm, we'll drink to get calmer. If we're depressed, we'll drink to anaesthetise.

I am lucky. I also discovered that I am one of the lucky ones. I am still breathing. I am here now. I have one life and I am going to make the most of what is left of it, whether it's one day or 40 years. I'm going to do it right now.

I can change my beliefs. One of the most important, if not THE most important thing anyone who drinks could learn is this: believing you can never stop drinking is just a belief. That's all it is. A false and limiting belief. And like all beliefs, they can be learned and unlearned. That's what I did. I changed my belief about alcohol. This book will show you how I did it.

STEPS YOU CAN TAKE

You might not think you have a problem with your alcohol consumption or your relationship with alcohol. But if you are reading this, the chances are that you are considering cutting back or stopping altogether.

STEP 1 – WRITE IT DOWN

Do what I did and write down an historical account of Alcohol & You. By writing down your story, you will soon build up a picture of your relationship with alcohol and whether you feel now is the right time to do something about it.

Get a piece of paper and split it into the following sections. Simply jot down what you can remember under each heading.

Your First Drink Ever

- Where were you?
- What was it?
- What did it taste like?
- Who were you with?
- Why did you drink it?
- What were the effects?

Your First Legal Drink (Over 18)

- Where were you?
- What was it?
- Who were you with?
- Why did you drink it?
- What were the effects?

Name The Times In Your Life When You Drank The Most

- Why did you drink?
- Do you find it easy or hard to stop drinking?

Name The Times In Your Life When You Drank The Least

- Why did you drink less?

People You Know

- Do you know any friends or family who have a problem with alcohol?
- Do you know anyone who has been seriously ill or even died as a result of alcohol?

Your Relationship With Alcohol Now

- Do you consider alcohol a problem?
- How much do you drink when you drink?
- How often do you drink?

Alcohol & The Future

- Do you want to drink less or stop drinking altogether?
- Why?

STEP 2 – START TO PUT A PLAN TOGETHER

If you want to take a break or stop drinking, the best course of action is to start to put a plan together to mastermind your escape. There are hundreds of tips and pointers throughout this book. I hope you enjoy reading about them as much as I have enjoyed living it.

KEY LEARNINGS

- How much you drink is NOT relevant to anybody else, only you, because it's all about you.
- I built a belief that drinking alcohol is cool, the normal thing to do.
- Believing you can never stop drinking is just a belief. That's all it is. A false and limiting belief.

CHAPTER 2
THE ALCOHOL DRINKERS' TRIBE
– THE ADT

Alcohol drinkers share several tribal characteristics, including a tendency to associate, identify and bond with other drinkers.

MY STORY

Anyone who drinks alcohol automatically joins what I call the 'Alcohol Drinkers' Tribe', or ADT, and anyone leaving the ADT automatically becomes a member of the 'Alcohol-Free Tribe', or AFT.

One of the biggest challenges on the journey to alcohol-free living is how to navigate leaving the ADT and how to deal with the reactions of drinkers because you left their tribe.

This tribalism metaphor is a great way to describe the sociology and psychology that plays out when someone decides to go alcohol-free and becomes a non-drinker. It's a great way of explaining what is going on both in the minds of the drinkers in the ADT and the ex-drinker who has decided to leave and join the AFT.

ALCOHOL & IDENTITY

Drinking became part of my identity. I am not sure of the exact point in my drinking relationship that this happened, but it definitely happened. It was probably early on. I think if someone is drinking regularly, whether that's every day or every weekend, then alcohol is defining them.

It was only when I finally admitted this to myself that I knew I could start to change my relationship with booze.

Alcohol was part of my identity, it was part of my belief system, just like politics and religion. If someone questioned my relationship with alcohol, I defended it, in some cases rigidly, just like I would a political standpoint or a religious view. This is why politics and religion are sometimes banned from dinner party talk as they inevitably lead to arguments because people can't help defending their viewpoints about their belief systems. This also explains why some drinkers get very agitated when someone they know stops drinking!

When you confuse what you believe with who you are, you tend only to hear things that support your view and shut out things that don't.

If someone told me that they'd 'stopped drinking because it's not fun any more, it makes me anxious, irritable, angry, moody and tired', I really didn't want to hear about it. It was far easier for me to just sum it all up quickly and put my alcohol-free friend, neighbour, relative or colleague in a box labelled 'has a drink problem' or something similar.

LEAVING THE TRIBE

In early human culture, I would have had to be a member of a tribe to survive. If I was banished from my tribe, I would almost certainly die. Lack of shelter, food and protection from wild beasts would be among the common causes of death.

We still keep with us this fear of leaving a tribe or tribes to which we belong. Today, however, the difference is that if we leave a tribe, in most cases, we don't die – we simply go and join another tribe.

When I was a member of the ADT, if another member told me they had decided that drinking was not for them and they were now living an alcohol-free life, my immediate assumption would have been that there must be something wrong with them.

Here are some of the beliefs and opinions that I have heard drinkers say about those who decide to go alcohol-free:

- They are an alcoholic.
- They must have a drink problem.
- They must be religious.
- They must have a career or a job that does not allow them to drink.
- It's just a temporary thing – they'll be drinking next week or in a month's time.

The reasons were very rarely based on the reality of what alcohol does to you, like...

They stopped because they realised it is:

- a dangerous drug that kills you.
- a poison.
- ruining their sleep.
- causing them regular anxiety attacks.

If I am truly honest with myself, and with the benefit of being alcohol-free for over a year, I believe I always knew deep down that alcohol was wrong, but I put that thought aside. In the early days when I was young and fit, I could get away with the trade-off between the feeling of being tipsy or drunk versus the payback hangover.

Whichever way I look at it, it was difficult to leave the tribe, but when the physical effects of hangovers, anxiety, sleep disruption and weight gain became too much, I really had to do something about it.

I probably spent 20 years wishing I could stop, but I really didn't know how to until I discovered the One Year No Beer Challenge (OYNB), which kick-started everything. To leave the ADT tribe, you need to find other people who think similarly. OYNB was that new tribe for me and through it, I now have access to online groups of thousands of like-minded people who are changing their relationship with alcohol.

I have no regrets about the past. What's the point in getting stressed over something you can't go back and change? At 56, I have at best 25 physically and mentally healthy years left.

It's time to look forward and say what is done is done. I'm in the AFT now. I'm not going to drink again. I'm going to enjoy the rest of my life.

WHAT I LEARNT

WHAT IS A TRIBE?

According to Professor Kevin deLaplante, an expert on tribalism, who runs the website *argumentninja.com*:

'A tribe is a social group with which we identify. It could be by religion, ethnicity, or for example a shared interest in a sports team.'

'Tribe members believe that judgements of their tribe are better, more justified, more reasonable and that judgements of those outside the tribe are compromised, are ignorant or they are worse people.'

The ADT is one of the world's biggest tribes with over 2.4 billion drinkers, based in every country on every continent.

In the UK alone, there are around 30 million drinkers, with an even mix of men and women of all ages. You can legally join the ADT at age 18 and most people stay members for life.

With such a large membership, it is common for tribe members to be from the same family. Most tribe members' friends and work colleagues are members. So, the average ADT member meets other members every day, through their family, friendships and the workplace. In short, it is hard to spend a day where you do not meet another member who reinforces the values of the ADT.

SHINE LIKE A BEACON

Most drinkers like to put people who have decided to stop drinking, or that don't drink, into boxes. That way they can deal with it quickly and get on with what they are used to, and that's continuing their drinking habit.

It's an easy way to deal with an issue that potentially questions their identity or belief system, and they need to comfort the discomfort the ex-drinker has exposed.

The act of leaving is a statement saying that 'the ex-drinker is now in control of their relationship with alcohol; it is not good for their health and well-being, and they have decided to move on and live a healthier and more fulfilling life.'

By stopping drinking, ex-drinkers become a beacon that glows and shines light on those around them. For those who continue to drink, this has the potential to highlight or put a focus on their relationship with alcohol.

In my experience, knowing someone who has stopped drinking leads members of the ADT to question their relationship with alcohol. Most will immediately decide that they would never stop drinking as they get too much pleasure out of it. Alcohol is their escape, their way of relaxing. Why on earth would they want to do what you are doing and leave the ADT? This is a delusion. A few might contemplate possibly joining you and leaving as well, but the fear of thinking they would not have fun any more keeps them in the ADT.

Realising that alcohol is slowly killing you, along with all the negative effects it has, is too close to home for ADT members – they firmly believe that alcohol is a fun, social pastime because this is what they have been brought up to think from day one by society.

STEPS YOU CAN TAKE

STEP 1 - HOW TRIBAL ARE YOU?

Ask yourself questions about the tribal characteristics of your relationship with alcohol. Take a guesstimate if you don't know the exact number. For example:

- What percentage of your friends are drinkers/non-drinkers?
- What percentage of your family are drinkers/non-drinkers?
- What percentage of people that you have contact with in your work environment are drinkers/non-drinkers?
- Overall, what percentage of everyone you know are drinkers/non-drinkers?
- Have you ever felt pressure to drink from friends, family, colleagues?
- If you stopped drinking, would you feel comfortable telling others, for example, your friends, family, colleagues? If not, why not?
- Are there any particular people you would not tell if you stopped drinking, and why?
- Are there any particular people you know would support you if you stopped drinking, and why?
- What do you think about people who have stopped drinking?

By doing this, you build up a picture of the people around you who drink and the influence they exert or may exert on you.

KEY LEARNINGS

- Alcohol drinkers share several tribal characteristics including a tendency to associate, identify and bond with other drinkers.

- Alcohol can become a major part of your identity.

- If you are drinking regularly, alcohol is defining you. Only when you admit it to yourself, can you truly start to change your relationship with it.

- When you confuse what you believe with who you are, you tend to only hear things that support your view and shut out things that don't.

- Most drinkers like to put people who have decided to stop drinking, or are teetotal, into boxes. It's an easy way to deal with an issue that potentially questions their identity or belief system.

CHAPTER 3
THE HABIT LOOP

What was the one thing I could give up in my life that would change everything and what was the one thing in my life that I had given up everything for? It was my relationship with alcohol.

MY STORY

When I started to look at myself, my actions, my values and my beliefs, I realised that I was living in a kind of self-made prison.

There is a beautiful world out there: a world where I am healthy, I am having fun, I am present, I am enjoying life, I have no anxiety, I am more compassionate, I am more empathetic, I am grateful and, above all, I am free. This is what the world was like when I was a child. I also experienced this world a few times over the years when I had stopped drinking for a few days. With hindsight, I would have loved to have stayed in this alcohol-free world but the pull of alcohol and the pressure to drink was always too much.

THE HABIT LOOP

Discovering the principles that make up habit loops helped me to understand how I could stop drinking, escape the clutches of alcohol and get on the pathway to freedom.

The psychologist Dan Siegel says that addiction 'is an illusion created by the brain'. I am convinced that drinking was etched into my brain, or neural pathways, and I firmly believed that it was a drug that I took to relax and unwind.

I believed alcohol was a relaxant which allowed my body to release dopamine as soon as I started to reach for the glass for the first sip. Dopamine is a neurotransmitter, meaning it sends signals from the body to the brain. This would give me an initial 'high'. This dopamine hit can come from a variety of places including chocolate, social media likes, exercise, or anything the brain associates with pleasure.

Craving alcohol in order to relax leads to a release of dopamine once the drinking ritual begins. This was giving me the 'high' feeling. So, if I kept doing this regularly, I got used to it and the 'high' feeling became less and less each time and so I needed more and more alcohol to feel the 'high'. This created a vicious cycle.

My habit loop went something like this...

CUE/TRIGGER/ REMINDER		ROUTINE/ HABIT		REWARD
6pm, end of working day	→	Drink glass of wine	→	Dopamine released

BREAKING THE HABIT LOOP

The million-dollar question was, could I break my alcohol habit loop? The answer was yes, and here's how.

I read that habits can prove difficult to break because the process is usually more complicated than simply quitting the behaviour or routine. However, change is possible.

I analysed the three parts of the habit loop and hatched a plan to keep it from playing on repeat.

I identified the specific cues that prompted me to drink – I already knew the routine and the reward!

The main cue for me was time. Specifically, 6pm weekdays or end of working day and lunch time on weekends.

NEW HABITS

After identifying this, I tried new behaviours instead of drinking, like drinking AF drinks or going for a walk. At first it was difficult and I needed to use an element of willpower. But over time, it started to get easier, and I eventually switched the habit.

I found out that the only way to break the alcohol habit loop is to replace the act of drinking with a new habit. In the first few days and weeks, I used the following 'new habits' to break the alcohol habit:

Talked to Others on an AF Journey – I joined an AF online community.

Read 'Quit Literature' – by this I mean the genre of books, which now includes this book! There are lots of great alcohol Quit Lit books. The ones I enjoyed the most were, *Alcohol Lied to Me* by Craig Beck, *This Naked Mind* by Annie Grace and *Freedom from Our Addictions* by Russell Brand. Although not directly alcohol related, I also enjoyed *Man's Search for Meaning* by Victor Frankl.

Lived A Healthier Lifestyle – having more energy made me want to do healthier things. In the first month, I set myself a goal of jogging 1km each day. I'd never jogged before. After 100 Days, I had halved my time.

Alcohol-Free (AF) Drinks – replacing an alcoholic drink with AF drinks. This is by far the best replacement in the first few weeks when cravings are at their highest and the habit loop is just starting to be broken.

Hobbies & Creativity – in the first months, I started learning lots of new things and building on hobbies I already had. I started learning the piano. I also took a lead guitar course, building on my rhythm playing, and learnt three or four new songs a week. I started writing and researching my family history. I also worked hard on my photography hobby, experimenting with many new techniques.

Kept a Journal – this is a great way of keeping a record of my new experiences and learnings. Over the year, I went back to these journals many times for reference. Nothing was lost.

Understanding habit loops allowed me to develop a plan. This was an important part of the way I stopped drinking.

WHAT I LEARNT

The concept of the habit loop was created by Charles Duhigg in his book *The Power of Habit: Why We Do What We Do in Life and Business*. There are three parts to the loop, which offer the key to deciphering how and why habits develop.

The first part or the cue, sometimes called the reminder, is the trigger that kicks off the habitual behaviour. Cues take the brain into a form of cruise control that prompts routine behaviours, or habits, that vary widely. They can take a lot of different forms and fall into several categories. The cues that triggered my habit of alcohol consumption were:

TYPE OF TRIGGER	SPECIFIC TRIGGERS/CUES
Location	The village pub, restaurants, cinema, train stations, trains, airports, planes
Time	6pm weekdays, lunchtime weekends, end of working day
Current Emotional State	Stressed, anxious, happy, celebratory
People Around Me	Work colleagues, clients, friends
My Last Action	After playing golf or playing any sport, after a long drive in the car

Some triggers were stronger than others. Probably the strongest one was 'time'. I would almost always crave a drink after the trigger of a day's completed work, so 6pm was a major trigger from Monday to Thursday, and a bit earlier on a Friday. On the weekend, the 'time' trigger was not so important. On Saturday and Sunday, location was a powerful trigger, particularly being in front of a large widescreen TV with a sports event just about to start, such as F1 at 1pm or a football match at 4pm.

The second part is the routine, the repeated behaviour or the habit. This might be something you're completely aware of, like taking a shower after waking up in the morning, or not aware of, like rubbing my knee while watching TV, which happens less consciously. I am only aware of this because my children get enormously wound up by it.

Habitual behaviours tend to happen automatically, though I probably made a conscious choice to pursue the action the first few times I did it. For example, if I've got some spare time sitting on a train or wherever I am and my phone is nearby, I'll look at Facebook or YouTube. This could turn into a bad habit.

For me, the alcohol habit was pouring a glass of wine or an ice-cold beer from my fridge. Over time, this routine became more automatic because of the third and final component of the habit loop – the reward.

The reward is what makes doing the routine worthwhile. Rewards reinforce routines and help keep habits alive.

This is the same for other habits. For example, joggers can experience a 'runner's high' through a dose of endorphins after a run – that's the reward. Gamblers experience similar chemical reactions in the brain when they gamble. Even the act of checking social media likes can give someone a release of endorphins.

CREATING NEW HABITS

You can never really eradicate habits 100% as the neurological patterns remain inside your brain. However, you can build new neurological patterns that override the old ones.

For instance, instead of drinking alcohol (the routine) when you have a craving brought on by, let's say, stress (the cue), you can go for a walk instead or have an AF drink leading to a reward of relaxation and feeling better. And similarly, if you want to start a new habit, all you need to do is create or identify a cue that will initiate a routine.

But identifying a cue and reward is often not enough to create a habit. Only when your brain begins to crave and expect this reward or a sense of accomplishment (the dopamine in the case of alcohol) does a new habit truly form. So only when you absolutely crave a walk, will walking truly become an ingrained habit. Research says it takes 60+ days to create a new habit. It worked for me.

STEPS YOU CAN TAKE

Work through the following three habit steps:

STEP 1 – GET TRIGGER HAPPY

Write down all the triggers and cues that made you crave that first drink, just like I did.

TYPE OF TRIGGER	LIST YOUR SPECIFIC TRIGGERS/CUES
Location	
Time	
Current Emotional State	
People Around Me	
My Last Action	

STEP 2 – LIST YOUR REWARDS

Make a list of what you think are the rewards, e.g. I feel relaxed, happy. You might find out that the rewards you think you get from drinking are not rewards at all!

STEP 3 – CREATE A LIST OF NEW HABITS

Create your own list of 'new habits' to replace the act of drinking and to break the alcohol habit loop, for example, have a hot bath, go for a walk, read a book, play a musical instrument.

KEY LEARNINGS

- Addiction is giving up everything for one thing. Recovery, or living an alcohol-free life, is giving up one thing for everything.

- There are three parts of the habit loop: the cue or trigger that kicks off the habitual behaviour; the routine or the habit or repeated behaviour; and the reward.

- The reward from alcohol is an immediate dose of a chemical called dopamine secreted into your body giving you a feeling of great pleasure.

- You can disrupt a habit by replacing the routine in the habit loop, while keeping the same cue and reward. That is how you 'break' habits. You keep the cue and the reward essentially the same; all you have to do is replace the routine.

- Understanding that your beliefs about alcohol could be wrong and need to be questioned is a critical part of the escape plan and the secret to becoming alcohol-free.

CHAPTER 4
ADDICTIVE BEHAVIOUR & BAD HABITS

I'm sure we have all said it jokingly, with a guilty smile, while buying a bottle of wine, or a lottery scratchcard, or a large bar of chocolate: 'It's my only vice!'

MY STORY

Once I stopped drinking, I had much more time to focus the spotlight on myself and I noticed that I had quite a few bad habits. By understanding how one habit is formed through a habit loop, I was able to see other habits more clearly.

I learnt that a growth mindset is the only way I could change my mind and break out of a habit loop, otherwise I would just spend years there!

Looking at my habits, I saw quickly that they were all interrelated. This fact only became apparent to me after I stopped drinking and was well on the road to healthy living and the new me. It was alcohol that was the root cause of my other 'bad' habits. This may or may not be true for you, but it certainly was for me. I know this because since I became alcohol-free, I have changed my relationship with all of them. Well, almost all of them!

Addiction is such a powerful and negative word. It conjures up, thanks to the movie industry, images of dirty, dark rooms, with drug users wrapping tourniquets around their arms to dilate their veins so that they can inject some nasty substance to take them to oblivion.

It also paints pictures in my mind of a gambler losing all his money and a drunk in an alleyway drinking from a bottle hidden in a brown paper bag. But, as I have discovered through reading and listening to numerous podcasts on my alcohol-free journey, addiction is part of our everyday lives. Most of us, if not all of us, are addicted to things or behaviours in some form.

COMMON HABITS & ADDICTIONS

A lot of people, including myself, do not know they are addicted to something. Many people drink far more than the government's recommended alcohol intake of 14 units per week but do not see their alcohol habit as an addiction. We don't like to admit weaknesses in ourselves, so denial is the first reaction.

My other bad habits, in addition to alcohol, were work, TV, social media, mobile phone usage and sugar. I say 'were' because I was able to use the same processes involved in stopping drinking alcohol to change my relationship with them.

I was not in the 'safe zone' for any of these because I answered 'yes' to the question: 'Is my usage causing me harm or damage?'

Here's a list of some of the most common addictions (only some affected me!):

- Alcohol
- Coffee
- Tobacco and nicotine
- Exercise
- Food

- Gambling
- Illegal & prescription drugs
- Mobile phones
- Plastic surgery
- Sex and pornography
- Shopping
- Social media
- Tanning
- TV
- Video games
- Work

WORK – THEN & NOW

I run my own marketing company and have done for over 20 years. Running a business can, and did, mean long hours. My office is next door to my house, situated in a village about 50 miles outside London. Although not technically working from home, the proximity to my workplace meant I was at my desk by 8am and there until 6pm every day. If I went to London, which was around six times a month, I would always go to the office first, so these days were even longer. Back at home, I would still check my emails well into the evening and first thing in the morning; sometimes, even when I woke up in the middle of the night. I was a workaholic, but I never realised I was until I stopped drinking and started looking at all aspects of my life and well-being.

If I was not putting in a full day's work, I felt anxious and guilty. A lot of this anxiety was caused by not being present in my mind, by not living in the now. It was caused by worrying about the future or getting stressed about past events, none of which I had any control over. Through mediation, however, I learnt how to free my mind to find space in between my thoughts. This amazing tool is so simple and so powerful. It is part of the secret to freeing myself from my addictions and bad habits. By learning how to be more present in my mind, I am less likely to get caught up in stories in my head or fall into reactive patterns of behaviour like arguing and making poor choices.

The biggest thing I learnt from mindfulness is how to build the 'window of reaction'. This is the time between stimulus and your reaction to a stimulus. For example, the stimulus could be, 'It's a sunny evening and I fancy a glass of wine'. One reaction might be to go ahead and have one; another, and the best course, would be to go and learn a new song on the guitar instead. If you can control the reaction to a stimulus, you are pretty much in control of your destiny.

I try to meditate at least once a day for around 10 to 15 minutes. This has had a massive effect on my whole life, including my attitude towards work, life balance and my old workaholism.

I now know that the only way to truly change is to change your mindset. Change the way you think about yourself. Meditation helps me to clear my mind of past or future thoughts and just think about what is now. This helps me think before I react. Einstein said: 'You can't solve a problem from the same state of mind that created it'. Change your mind; change your story; change your life.

I now go to the office at around 9.30am, after I have completed my morning walk, showered and had breakfast. Being fitter and having more energy means I am more productive. I can now do in three hours what previously took me six. My brain feels sharper, quicker, more efficient, partly because I have not had a hangover for 18 months. Also, being more present means I focus on what's happening now. My mind is not wandering to the past or the future. It's reunited with my body, here in the present – the only place where things happen.

TV, SOCIAL MEDIA & MOBILE – THEN & NOW

In my drinking days, I would think nothing of spending the whole evening in front of the TV, sometimes to the early hours, binge-watching some multi-part series with a glass in hand. The amount of time I wasted doing this is now unthinkable – probably 25 to 30 hours a week, every week. So, well over 1,000 hours a year. I would now call this a bad habit.

I have now completely changed my relationship with TV, like I did with alcohol. I watch two or three films a month. The scary thing is that I have watched a few films for a second time, this time without the influence of alcohol, and they are so much better now. It's like I am watching a different film!

Social media and mobile phone usage followed a similar pattern. Over 90% of my social media usage was through my mobile phone. I was checking my email every 15 minutes, as well as viewing Facebook, TikTok and YouTube.

The skills I learnt to crush alcohol have been invaluable in addressing these other habits. It is all about understanding the habit loop. Once you know what triggers your habit, you can replace that habit with something else. So instead of sitting in front of the TV, I now do one of my hobbies each evening – as well as writing this book!

I limit myself to certain times of the day when I allow myself to use the phone and social media. One of the best things I did was to turn off notifications on all apps. I had no idea how addictive notifications can be. My phone was bleeping every few seconds, which meant I was looking at it and getting caught up in social media and email.

Once you turn off notifications, you are in charge. You go to the phone when you want to. It does not call you any more to tell you someone has just posted something on LinkedIn.

Stopping drinking completely changes your life. It gave me back the time that I was throwing away, in front of a TV screen, numbed by ethanol. When I speak to others who are on the alcohol-free journey, they all agree that one of the major surprises is the sheer amount of time you have and the things you can do with it.

SUGAR & SALT – THEN & NOW

Last, but not least, I do have a sweet tooth and was partial to salty snacks. However, I am very pleased to announce that since I stopped drinking, my intake of salty snacks is almost zero. I always associated them with drinking alcohol; they literally went hand in hand. So, it was easy to stop eating them.

I still eat sweet things in the evenings so am keeping an eye on this. The fact that I now walk over 9km every day, plus other exercise, means that my whole mindset has changed and I don't look at sweet things like I used to. I now understand that they could be bad for me if eaten excessively. So, an occasional piece of cake, biscuit or chocolate bar is still allowed.

WHAT I LEARNT

UNDERSTANDING ADDICTION

According to the drug & alcohol resources, support & guidance website *Recovery Connection*, addiction is defined as obsessive thinking and compulsive need for drugs, alcohol, food, sex or anything, despite the resulting negative consequences. Addiction includes the development of tolerance combined with withdrawal symptoms.

Addiction develops over time and usually begins with misuse, moving toward abuse and resulting in addiction.

STEPS YOU CAN TAKE

STEP 1 – MAKE A LIST OF YOUR HABITS

These could include: coffee; tobacco and nicotine; alcohol; sex and pornography; illegal or prescription drugs; gambling.

Then write down the average amount of time you spend on, or the amount you consume of, each.

STEP 2 – ARE YOU IN THE SAFE ZONE?

To see if you are in the 'safe zone', ask yourself the question: 'Is my usage of any of these potential addictions causing me harm or damage?'

If it is, then maybe it's time to do something about it!

KEY LEARNINGS

- Addiction is defined as obsessive thinking and a compulsive need for drugs, alcohol, food, sex or anything, despite the resulting negative consequences.

- It was alcohol that was the root cause of many of my other bad habits.

- The nature of addiction makes it difficult to recognise the addiction in oneself.

- Einstein said: 'You can't solve a problem from the same state of mind that created it'.

- The skills I have learnt to crush alcohol can be used to address other bad habits.

- Understanding the habit loop is key. Once you know what triggers your habit, you replace the habit with something else.

- Stopping drinking completely changed my life. It gave me the time back that I was throwing away in front of a TV screen, numbed by ethanol. I was astonished by the sheer amount of time I gained and the things I could do with it.

CHAPTER 5
CURIOSITY SAVED THIS CAT – ALCOHOL FACTS

During the first few weeks of my alcohol-free journey, I started to look in depth at the statistics regarding alcohol – it was mind-blowing. These facts played a huge part in helping to convince me that things had to change.

MY STORY

There's a saying that 'curiosity killed the cat'. Essentially, it's telling you be wary of being curious. If you are curious, it could cost you your life. It's saying, keep in line and don't ask too many questions. It's one of those sayings that was passed down to me as a child, even though I'm not sure where I heard it. But this belief was hanging around somewhere in my subconscious mind. It is an incredibly powerful belief and one that I had carried around with me all my life.

One of the changes I made was to get rid of my limiting beliefs and this one had to go. I prefer now 'curiosity saved the cat' – that way you get to question things with a more open mind without the fear of death or something bad hanging over you.

Put very simply, I got curious about booze.

It is really only the first drink or the first few seconds that makes you feel 'good'. It's only the first sip of the first drink that gives you the 'best' whoosh feeling. And if you are honest with yourself, it only lasts 10-20 seconds. I began to see alcohol as a trade. Every time I drank it, I was trading away my life. Take the weekend as an example. EVERY Friday night, I effectively traded my weekend for the initial 20-second whoosh that the first of a few drinks gave me. What an idiot!

Now, well into my second year alcohol-free, I have had over 100 hangover-free weekend mornings and I completely appreciate the weekends. The days are now gone when I would get up after 9am with a hangover, eat fried and junk food most of Saturday to feel better, and would almost definitely have another drink to feel normal again.

WHAT I LEARNT

DOPAMINE – HOW ALCOHOL GIVES YOU A HIGH

To understand how alcohol pulls you in, you need to understand what's happening medically. That can be summed up in one word: dopamine.

When you drink alcohol, your brain releases dopamine, which makes you feel good. Your brain, therefore, assumes this is a reward and encourages you to repeat this behaviour, even though the alcohol may not be the healthiest choice for your body.

It's dopamine that gives you the initial high or whoosh feeling. By drinking alcohol, you are interfering with your body's dopamine system.

Interacting with the pleasure and reward centre of your brain, dopamine – along with other chemicals like serotonin, oxytocin and endorphins – plays a vital role in how happy you feel. In addition to your mood, dopamine also affects movement, memory and focus. Healthy levels of dopamine drive you to seek and repeat pleasurable activities, while low levels can have an adverse physical and psychological impact.

When the brain has a healthy level of dopamine, you feel good. Your motivation increases. You're productive. You plan well. You learn quickly. You're driven, excited about life, focused and attentive. Healthy levels of dopamine can make you more sociable and extroverted. Dopamine also helps increase your empathy for others, making you more willing to adapt to others' needs.

All of these attributes help produce the pleasurable feelings dopamine is known for.

ALCOHOL AND LOW LEVELS OF DOPAMINE

Abnormally low levels of dopamine are associated with high alcohol consumption and can cause physical and mental impairments because this major body chemical controls so many body functions. Low dopamine has been linked to impairments such as: anxiety, addiction, behavioural disturbances, brain fog, mental health disorders, mood swings, delusional behaviour, depression, feelings of hopelessness, low self-esteem, lack of motivation, suicidal thoughts or thoughts of self-harm, low sex drive and psychosis. Any of these sound familiar?

A release of dopamine is what tells the brain whether an experience was pleasurable enough to experience again. When there is a lack of dopamine, it can cause people to change their behaviours in ways that will help release more of this chemical. They will pursue activities that trigger their reward centre, even if these activities are harmful or taboo. They may seek illicit drugs or alcohol or engage in other harmful, addictive behaviours. An imbalance of dopamine can create an unhealthy reward system response in the brain.

The genetics department of the University of Utah explains that 'all addictive drugs affect brain pathways involving reward, that is, the dopamine system in the reward pathway'. The impact that drugs and alcohol have on the natural reward centre is more intense than is naturally found in the body. This over-stimulation may, according to university researchers, 'decrease the brain's response to natural rewards' and may result in a person's inability to feel pleasure except as triggered by the abused substance.

Because dopamine is the chemical that drives us to seek positive experiences and avoid negative ones, when this reward system is damaged, human behaviour patterns may change to seek out harmful situations and substances as a means of pleasure.

WHAT DOES ALCOHOL DO TO YOUR BODY?

Here are just a few of the lies I told myself everyday:

- Alcohol relaxes me.
- It makes me a fun person. I can't have fun without a drink.
- One drink is not going to hurt me.
- It makes me sleep better.

What does it really do? Here are just a few of the bad things:

ANXIETY & DEPRESSION	It depresses the central nervous system. It sedates you. Feeling of not being present. Worrying about the future or fretting over the past. Daytime sleepiness, depression, low performance. Suicidal thoughts.
HEALTH	Liver failure, diabetes, obesity, heart disease and cancer. To name a few.
SLEEP	Alcohol leads to real sleep problems including waking up in the middle of the night to go the loo. Not being able to go back to sleep because of the anxiety it induces. Less Rapid Eye Movement (REM) sleep – this is when the deepest stage of sleep occurs. Nightmares, leading to a restless night.
SWEATS	It makes you sweat.

JUDGEMENT	It affects judgement – drinkers become more accident-prone and have less mental alertness.
HANGOVERS	It leads to physical and mental fatigue, ruining the next day.
REGRET	Causes regret over so many things done while under its influence, from over-eating mindlessly to ruined relationships.
LOW SELF-WORTH	Alcohol can lead to a feeling of low self-worth. Lots of shame and self-loathing over, for example, not setting a good example to your children. Also a feeling of failure and guilt that you have let yourself and loved ones down.
CIRCADIAN RHYTHM	As the sedative effect wears off, alcohol consumption can interfere with your circadian rhythm, the internal master clock in your brain. It helps sync your body's functions and activities. The CR is a 24-hour cycle that includes physiological and behavioural rhythms, including sleeping, appetite, body temperature, alertness and reaction times.
BEHAVIOUR CHANGE	Alcohol can result in aggressive, abusive behaviour.

Alcohol harms people through mental health problems, liver disease, cancer, economic difficulties, relationship breakdown, loss of livelihood and so much more. It can affect any one of us, from any walk of life.

This harm doesn't end with the drinker. Each person who drinks too much is part of a family and/or a community who feel the effects too through, for example, frequent use of emergency services, drink-driving, violence or neglect.

STEPS YOU CAN TAKE

STEP 1 – WHAT ARE YOUR EXISTING BELIEFS ABOUT ALCOHOL?

Create a table with two columns. In column one, write down your existing beliefs about alcohol. For example, they may all be positive: it's fun; the amount I drink won't hurt me; it helps me sleep; it helps me relax.

STEP 2 – GET CURIOUS

Get curious about alcohol. Read as much alcohol 'Quit Lit' as possible and see both sides of the argument. Find out what others are saying.

Don't believe that the drinks industry, which spends billions annually promoting the 'benefits' of alcohol, is telling you the truth!

Start seeing alcohol for what it really is. *Alcohol Change* UK has some great facts and figures and is a great start point.

Return to the table you created in STEP 1 and write down in column two your beliefs about alcohol now you have become curious.

Is it time to change your beliefs about alcohol?

Only you can make this decision.

STEP 3 – START TRIGGERING YOUR DOPAMINE FROM OTHER SOURCES

The good news is that there are many ways you can naturally increase your dopamine levels, without drinking alcohol.

When you stop drinking and break your alcohol habit, it does not mean you can never again get that 'high' feeling alcohol gives you. In fact, I get natural highs from just living an alcohol-free life. The longer you go into the journey, the more it happens.

You can naturally boost dopamine levels by:

- **Listening to music.** A small study investigating the effects of music on dopamine found that people who listened to instrumental songs that gave them an emotional response, had a 9% increase in brain dopamine levels.
- **Engaging in healthy lifestyle practices.** Exercise, meditation, gardening, reading or even playing with a pet.
- **Maintaining a healthy diet.** Foods that are rich in tyrosine, like almonds, eggs, fish and chicken, are especially good for boosting dopamine levels.
- **Spending more time outdoors.** Science consistently shows that low exposure to sunshine can reduce levels of dopamine. Similarly, increased sunlight exposure can help raise levels.

KEY LEARNINGS

- Alcohol harms people through mental health problems, liver disease, cancer, economic difficulties, relationship breakdown, loss of livelihood and so much more.
- It can affect any one of us, from any walk of life.
- It is really only the first drink or the first few seconds that is making you feel 'good'. It's only the first sip of the first drink that gives you the 'whoosh' feeling.
- When you drink alcohol, your brain releases dopamine which makes you feel good. Your brain, therefore, assumes this is a reward and encourages you to repeat this behaviour, even though the alcohol may not be the healthiest choice for your body.
- Though alcohol use is harmful, the brain only recognises it as a source of pleasure and does not seek to stop the behaviour. The person's mind now sees alcohol use as a pleasurable experience, even if this is an irrational choice for their overall health.

- The good news is that there are many ways you can naturally increase your dopamine levels without drinking alcohol.

- When you stop drinking and break your alcohol habit it does not mean you can never again get that high feeling alcohol gives you. You can naturally boost dopamine levels from lots of different activities, including listening to music, engaging in healthy lifestyle practices, maintaining a healthy diet and spending more time outdoors.

- If you believe the facts about alcohol, and there is no reason why you should not, then why would you want to carry on drinking, other than you like dancing with the devil?

CHAPTER 6
HOW SAUCY ARE YOU?

Everyone is different when it comes to alcohol. Each of us has our own special relationship with booze. In this chapter, you get the opportunity to categorise yourself and take a new test I created called the How Saucy Are You? Test. You can use this to measure how much control you have over your relationship with alcohol.

MY STORY

What type of drinker are you?

An occasional drinker – those who like a wee dram, a tiny tot or a naughty nip, not very often and on your terms.

A heavy drinker – those who feel the need for a lunchtime snifter, a daily bracer or a crafty half that becomes a dirty dozen; you have become the lush on the lash.

Or are you somewhere in the middle? – you are in control, well, at least you believe you are. The closest you'll get to a six-pack is in the off-licence.

Over the 35 years that I drank, I'd been called a few things related to my drinking. I'd also called myself a few things!

I did not fit perfectly into any of the stereotypical profiles but I could relate in part to the *Home Drinker* and *Secret Drinker* and at times I could be a bit of a *Bar Fly*, which are all described below in more detail.

So, let's jump straight in, cards on table. My *How Saucy Are You? Test* score was 64%, putting me firmly in the drinking-too-much end of the spectrum.

TAKE THE HOW SAUCY ARE YOU? TEST

The *How Saucy Are You? Test* is not designed to be an all-encompassing analysis of drinker types, but it does allow you to step outside yourself and see your drinking habit from different perspectives. It will also help you to learn how to manage your relationship with alcohol. It's a lot easier to deal with the problem if you know what you are up against.

The *How Saucy Are You? Test* measures how potentially 'out of control' your relationship with alcohol is. It will give you an 'out of control' score between 0 and 100%.

Zero is teetotal – you don't drink.

Up to 20% – you're likely to be an occasional drinker.

21-40% – you're likely to be a regular drinker.

41-60% – you're likely to be already thinking about changing your relationship with alcohol.

Anything over 60% – you're in the danger zone and need to take a serious look at your relationship with drinking. It could be massively affecting your health.

Alcohol can make us deluded. You might think you are in control of your drinking, when the reality is that you are on the brink of it developing into a serious health problem.

By gaining a better understanding of how you see your relationship with alcohol and comparing this to how friends or family see it, you can gain real insight into whether you have a problem, or potential problem, with the sauce.

For the best insight, compare the score you give yourself with the score friends or family members give you.

HOW SAUCY ARE YOU? TEST QUESTIONNAIRE

Score each question between 0 and 10. For example, score yourself as follows:

- never/no time – 0
- very little time – 1 or 2
- a small amount of time – 3 or 4
- an average amount of time – 5 or 6
- a lot of the time – 7 or 8
- all or most of the time – 9 or 10

QUESTIONS	YOUR SCORE 0-10
How often do you crave alcohol?	
How often do you consume alcohol and spend time recovering from its aftermath?	
Do you have difficulties controlling how often you drink?	
Do you give up activities to drink instead?	
Do you drink to feel 'normal'?	
When you drink alcohol, do you become angry?	
When you drink alcohol, does your judgement become clouded?	
When you drink alcohol, do you experience memory loss?	
When you drink alcohol, does it interfere with fulfilling regular life obligations?	
When you drink alcohol, do you damage your relationships and social interactions?	
SCORE*	-- / 100

*Percentage your relationship with alcohol is potentially 'out of control'.

HOW SAUCY ARE YOU? TEST: CLASSIFICATION

OCCASIONAL DRINKER	LIGHT REGULAR DRINKER	REGULAR DRINKER	SERIOUS DRINKER	HEAVY DRINKER
1-20%	21-40%	41-60%	61-80%	81-100%

WHAT I LEARNT

When analysing my relationship with drink I started to pull together a list of other terms I had heard or seen, which classify drinkers based on their relationship with alcohol. These are based on level of control and are set out in the table below.

I decided to write down all these stereotypes and came up with the following list. It's by no means exhaustive and is meant as a rough-and-ready way to classify people. Can you see yourself? You may be a cross between one or more types.

Towards the end of my drinking days, I had become mainly a *Home Drinker*, drinking mostly at home, or after a few drinks in the pub, I would end up drinking a bottle of wine at home.

TYPES OF DRINKER

TYPES OF DRINKER	DEPENDENCY	CORE ATTRIBUTE
BAR FLY	Possibly	Tends to drink alone at the bar. Keen to have small talk with bar staff and other drinkers. Gives the impression to the outside world that they are a moderate drinker.
BINGE DRINKER	Highly Likely	Normally a weekend Friday/Saturday night boozer. Can really put it away, up to the four bottles of wine or 15+ pints but they really pay for it the next day with a 'mother' of hangovers.
DRINKER'S DRINKER	Highly Likely	Always laughing. Always getting the drinks in. Guaranteed to be at all drinking occasions. Likely to be an organiser making sure everyone comes along to the party and everything they organise is based around booze. Makes sure everyone has a drink. They never have an empty glass.
HOME DRINKER	Highly Likely	Do most of their drinking at home. Or, after a few drinks in the pub, will end up drinking a bottle of wine at home – maybe more. Ends the night with a nightcap.
OCCASIONAL DRINKER	No	This person really can take it or leave it. At one extreme, there is the *Very Light Occasional Drinker* who might have a drink three or four times a year – maybe a glass of wine or champagne at Christmas, maybe at a wedding. You can count on one hand the times they drink during a year. They hardly ever get drunk and if they do, it's after two or three drinks. At the other end of the spectrum, the *Occasional Drinker* may drink a few times each month and very rarely loses control. By their nature, they are not regular drinkers.

PACK DRINKER	Possibly	This drinker rarely drinks alone and feels at home when drinking with a group of people.
PROBLEM DRINKER	Yes	They realise that their drinking is a problem. They really don't know how to deal with it. Everything in their life is based on alcohol. All roads lead to alcohol – friends, bar in their home, etc. Some want to quit but don't know how to or are worried of failing as they think it will be too hard.
PROSECCO DRINKER	Possibly	Normally drink in groups but are also known to put a bottle away while watching TV or talking to friends on the phone.
THE QUITTER	Highly Likely	Is normally a *Problem Drinker* who wants to stop forever or have more control over their relationship with alcohol and become just an *Occasional Drinker*.
SECRET DRINKER	Highly Likely	Drinks at home a lot. People close to them don't know the full extent of the problem. Happy to drink alone.
TEENAGE DRINKER	No, but could easily become	Drinking is a rite of passage. They're saying to everybody else – I'm an adult; I'm grown-up; I'm living on my own; I'm drinking like the adults did when I lived at home. They've learnt from advertisements, movies, their parents, that alcohol is part of growing up. Likely to have a drink on their 18th birthday. Under 18, will probably try to get into pubs pretending they're older. Their parents or guardians may even buy them a drink when they're 16/17 sitting in a beer garden. They don't really care about the physical and mental effects because they're young, their bodies are stronger, and it doesn't affect them as much as it would an older person. If they have a hangover, they can cope with it.

WEEKEND ONLY	Possibly	This type is a form of *Binge Drinker*.

STEPS YOU CAN TAKE

STEP 1 – TAKE THE 'HOW SAUCY ARE YOU?' TEST.

Is it what you expected?

Ask a close friend, partner, family member to score you as well. Compare your scores.

Ask yourself the question: Do you want to carry on as you are or make a change?

The decision is yours!

STEP 2 – WHAT TYPE OF DRINKER ARE YOU?

Take a look at the Types of Drinker profiles above. Can you see yourself? You may be a cross between one or more types.

KEY LEARNINGS

- Everyone is different when it comes to alcohol. Each of us has our own special relationship with booze.

- By gaining a better understanding of the different types of drinker, it's easier to identify how alcohol may be affecting you and help you to identify and learn how to manage your relationship with it.

CHAPTER 7
ALCOHOLOMETER – HOW MUCH PURE ALCOHOL DO YOU DRINK?

We all know it's poison. In fact, we even have a saying when offering someone a drink: 'What's your poison?'

According to medical experts, if you drank around half a pint of 100% undiluted alcohol you would almost certainly die.

Armed with that information, would you do that? Of course you wouldn't... or would you?

MY STORY

When I got curious about alcohol, I started to work out how much neat or pure alcohol I was drinking.

Towards the end of my drinking days, each week I was drinking roughly: half a bottle of spirits (ABV 40%), 7 bottles of wine (ABV 12.5%) and 6 pints of beer (ABV 5%).

By doing a very quick calculation, using the amount of alcohol content called Alcohol By Volume, or ABV, printed on the side of the bottle, I concluded my neat alcohol intake per week was: 140ml from spirits, 656ml from wine and 199ml from beer. Total 995ml – let's call it a litre per week. That's 52 litres or over 100 pints a year!

Who on earth would want to drink 52 litres of neat, undiluted poison each year? That's equivalent to a whole bath of poison. Over 30 years, that added up to 1,500 litres of pure alcohol. The answer was 'Me', but things were about to change for good.

THE ALCOHOLOMETER

I created the Alcoholometer as a guide to calculate the amount of neat or pure alcohol I was drinking.

BEER

Let's take beer for example. Beer and lagers are around 4-6% ABV. Some are stronger, even up to 10% ABV, and some weaker. That simply means that if you had a glass of beer containing a pint (568ml) of 5% ABV beer, it would contain approximately 28ml of neat alcohol. This means that for every 20 pints of beer with a 5% ABV you drink, you would consume one pint of neat alcohol. WOW! Remember half a pint of neat alcohol drunk straight down would kill you.

If I put a pint of neat alcohol in front of a beer drinker, they would not drink it. But they are quite happy to consume the alcohol diluted. I knew a few people who could drink 20 pints in a session!

Let's dig a bit deeper. Let's say you drink a couple of pints after work, Monday to Thursday. On the weekend, you let your hair down and have five pints on Friday, and maybe an afternoon session with some satellite sports on Saturday, consuming six pints. Then on Sunday, a 'hair-of-the-dog' pint with your lunch. That's 20 pints, or one pint of neat alcohol. If you did that every week you would consume 52 pints of neat alcohol a year just through drinking beer. That's 29.5 litres. Based on 5% ABV.

WINE

What about wine? Roughly, wines are 12-13.5% ABV. Some are stronger, even up to 15% ABV, and some weaker. This means that for every eight 750ml bottles of wine with a

12.5% ABV you drink, you consume one 750ml bottle of neat alcohol. Another WOW!

So, someone drinking a bottle of wine per night at 12.5% ABV would consume 365 bottles a year equating to 34.21 litres of neat alcohol. That's crazy. Why the hell would you do that to your body and your loved ones? Surely you owe yourself, and them, more than that!

SPIRITS

And finally, spirits, for those that live in the fast lane! This is one of the closest ways you can get to drinking neat alcohol. An average bottle of spirits contains 700ml, roughly 14 doubles. Let's say you have a couple of doubles as a nightcap each evening. That's a bottle per week or 52 bottles a year. Now, each bottle contains 40% neat alcohol or 280ml (roughly half a pint). So, each year, you would be drinking 14.56 litres of neat alcohol based on a couple of nightcaps each evening!

	BEER	WINE	SPIRITS
AMOUNT CONSUMED	20 pints per week for a year	1 x 75cl bottle of wine every night	2 x double nightcaps a night
ABV	5% ABV	12.5% ABV	40% ABV
AMOUNT OF PURE ALCOHOL CONSUMED IN A YEAR	29.54 litres	34.21 litres	14.56 litres

When put like this, it became easy for me to start to accept that drinking alcohol was a form of suicide I was putting myself through. I had to stop.

This is exactly the type of information that convinced my unconscious mind that alcohol is bad.

This is how I started to change my beliefs about alcohol. I looked at the hard facts. I looked at the reality of what I was doing to myself.

In the STEPS YOU CAN TAKE section below you can use the Alcoholometer to work out your own pure alcohol consumption.

WHAT I LEARNT

HISTORICAL FACT – PROOF VS ABV

In the 18th Century, the alcohol content of alcoholic drinks was expressed as 'proof', which came about because British sailors were paid with money as well as rum. In order to ensure that the rum was not diluted with water, it was 'proofed' by mixing gunpowder with it and setting it on fire. If the gunpowder failed to ignite, it meant that the rum was diluted with excess water.

These measures can be a bit confusing because they differ around the world! In the USA, proof to alcohol by volume is a ratio of 1:2. So, a beer which has 4% ABV is 8% Proof. In the UK, ABV to proof is a ratio of 4:7. So, multiplying ABV content with a factor of 1.75 would provide the 'proof' of the drink.

WHAT WE ARE TOLD

Every bottle, can, box or carton of alcohol sold or poured must have its ABV (Alcohol By Volume) percentage written on it. This is so the drinker is aware that what they are drinking contains alcohol, and the ABV tells them how much. The government in its wisdom decided that it would be a good idea to warn people about the amount of alcohol contained in their favourite beverages.

But it does not tell us that what we are about to drink has a similar chemical formula to car fuel!

THE ALCOHOLOMETER & GOVERNMENT ADVICE

The alcohol served up in alcoholic beverages is called ethyl alcohol or ethanol. Consuming it alone can cause coma and death.

According to the Drinkaware website, the Chief Medical Officer's guideline for both men and women states that to keep health risks from alcohol to a low level, it is safest not to drink more than 14 units a week on a regular basis.

So, let's have a closer look using the Alcoholometer. If you drank roughly 14 units a week, every week of the year, you would drink the following amounts of neat or pure alcohol:

DRINK TYPE	WEEKLY	NO. OF WEEKLY UNITS	ANNUAL EQUIVALENT VOLUME	ANNUAL EQUIVALENT PURE ALCOHOL
Beer (4% ABV)	6 x Pints (568ml)	13.6	312 x 568ml Pints x 4%	7.01 litres
Beer (5% ABV)	8 x Bottles (330ml)	13.2	416 x 330ml Bottles x 5%	6.86 litres
Cider (4.5% ABV)	5 x Pints (568ml)	12.8	260 x 568ml Pints x 4.5%	6.65 litres
Wine (13% ABV)	6 x Glasses (175ml)	13.7	312 x 175ml Glasses x 13%	7.01 litres
Champagne (12% ABV)	9 x Glasses (125ml)	13.5	468 x 125ml Glasses x 12%	7.02 litres
Spirits (40% ABV)	7 x Glasses (50ml)	14	26 x 700ml Bottles x 40%	7.28 litres

STEPS YOU CAN TAKE

STEP 1 – WORK OUT THE UNITS YOU DRINK

If you want to understand how many units you are drinking per week, you can work out your own alcohol unit intake on the calculator at https://www.drinkaware.co.uk/facts/alcoholic-drinks-and-units/low-risk-drinking-guidelines

One unit is 10ml of pure alcohol. Because alcoholic drinks come in different strengths and sizes, units are a good way of telling how strong your drink is. It's not as simple as: one drink, one unit.

The new alcohol unit guidelines are equivalent to six pints of average-strength beer, or six 175ml glasses of average-strength wine, per week.

STEP 2 – USE THE ALCOHOLOMETER

Work out how much neat alcohol you are consuming (see the Alcoholometer tables in the appendix).

Write it down and put it on a sticky note on your fridge door. Every time you go to the fridge for a glass of wine or a beer, it will be a reminder.

KEY LEARNINGS

- The alcohol served up in alcoholic beverages is called ethyl alcohol or ethanol.

- Ethanol is most commonly used in alcoholic beverages. It is also used in many household and workplace items, including varnishes, nail polish remover, perfumes, biofuel, gasoline additive, preservative for biochemical samples, medicines, household cleaning products, beauty products and various solvents.

- Consuming ethanol alone can cause coma and death. According to medical experts, if you drank around half a pint of 100% undiluted ethanol you would almost certainly die.

- A major component of being able to change my beliefs about alcohol was through the Alcoholometer. Calculating my alcohol consumption this way left me nowhere to hide.

- Someone drinking a couple of pints of 5% ABV beer each day would consume 730 pints a year equating to 20.73 litres of neat alcohol.

- Someone drinking a bottle of wine per night at 12.5% ABV would consume 365 bottles a year equating to 34.21 litres of neat alcohol.

- A couple of double spirits as a nightcap each evening – a bottle per week or 52 bottles a year – is the equivalent of drinking 14.56 litres of neat alcohol.

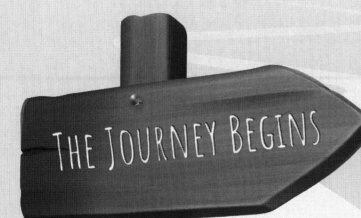

The First Few Days

THE JOURNEY BEGINS: THE FIRST FEW DAYS

Getting past the first few days can be the hardest part of the journey, but with the right mindset it doesn't have to be.

This section looks at the positive psychology approach to stopping drinking. Yes, there is a bit of white knuckle willpower needed, but if you manage it correctly, it becomes an enjoyable, fun journey. With the right mindset, the journey gets better every day and never stops delivering for your well-being.

This book is not just about stopping drinking. It's also about finding happiness and contentment. It's about taking a big, gigantic look at yourself to understand what's wrong, and to change it for the good. I look at my beliefs about alcohol. I look at why I wanted – and needed – to stop drinking.

I then delve into my values, beliefs and purpose, and show you how I changed my story.

I changed the way I look at the world. It changed my life and made me feel like I'm in my 20s again.

CHAPTER 8
GET WISE ABOUT YOUR WHYS

On the surface, this book is about stopping drinking. But it's much bigger than that. It's about how you can change your beliefs, learn to believe in yourself, and achieve anything you want to do through a few simple changes. The answer is already in your mind. You just need to discover where to find it.

MY STORY

The first thing I did at the start of my alcohol-free journey was to write down my 'whys', or the reasons why I am doing this in the first place; the reasons why I am going on this life-changing journey.

I looked at these 'whys' as part of my goals. The author Napoleon Hill defines a goal as, 'a dream with a deadline'. I love that. Goals helped my brain select the people, resources and ideas that I needed to live my dreams and realise my 'whys'.

The *One Year No Beer Challenge* was a great help and catalyst for me because it helped me find the path. In the early days, it helped me structure my journey, by providing a daily video, which landed in my inbox just after 6am every morning. This reminded me of what day of the challenge I was on, together with some words of wisdom and a reflection for the day.

TIME TO CHANGE

My drinking had made me overweight and unfit. I had sleep problems and didn't have the best of relationships with those close to me.

I hoped that by stopping drinking I would become healthier, happier, lighter, freer and have better relationships. I believed I would have more time and more money, saved from not spending it on alcohol.

Things really had to change, as I now firmly believed that if I continued along the path I was on, I would face drastic health implications and quite possibly an early death. Nice!

Above everything else, by a long way, there was one thing that needed to change. Initially, I wrote in my journal, 'I must stop drinking in the evenings and on Sunday during the day'. There was still something in me trying to hang on to the occasional drink. Who was I kidding? I thought about this, crossed it out and then wrote, 'I'd like to stop drinking forever.' This was my dream. I now needed to give it a deadline and that came in the form of the *One Year No Beer Challenge*. At the start, thinking that I could stop drinking for a whole year was just a dream. But I knew that if I did that, I would be free from alcohol forever.

IDENTIFYING MY WHYS

I thought about the things I could achieve, now I had the motivation, and wrote down in my journal, '*In the short term, lose one stone (6kg) in weight and run one mile (1.6km) without stopping. In the longer term, lose five stone (30kg) and be able to run five miles (8km).*' I was over 17 stone (108kg) and could only run 200 yards (182m) without stopping to catch my breath. So this was a big challenge for me.

Here are my original 'whys' from Day One of my daily journal. These are the exact words I scribbled down:

To be healthier – to minimise risk of cancer, liver problems, heart disease, etc.

To lose weight – to look better and be able to wear nicer clothes.

To not look like I am a drinker!

To have a better and more fulfilling relationship with my family – my wife, my children and my mother.

I then split these 'whys' or goals into short-term and long-term, as follows:

SHORT-TERM WHYS/GOALS	LONG-TERM WHYS/GOALS
Feel better	Sleep better, stop snoring
Better skin	Look better
Less stressed	Be calm and collected

When I stopped drinking alcohol, a whole new world opened up for me. I have more energy, more time – loads more time! I want to learn more. I want to live life to the full.

If you stopped people in the street and asked them what their goals are, you'd quickly find out that most people do not have any. They get up every day without a plan; just mindlessly getting on with their lives with their heads down accepting their lot. Not me.

Imagine asking the captain of a ship, 'Where are you heading?' and they say, 'I don't know.' This is the same as having no goals to aim for, no targets. You end up rudderless in a sea of other people's dreams and ambitions.

I now had a shedload of time on my hands and so I started to fill it with the stuff I'd always wanted to do but never had time to because I was too busy drinking alcohol most nights and weekends, believing I was having a great time and relaxing. Can you see the irony?

TYPES OF GOAL

I focussed on types of goal. This is a great way to get a plan down on paper. You'll be surprised what can fall out of this and quickly become a reality.

MY GOAL TYPES	MY GOALS OR MY PROJECTS	TIMING
Physical Well-being	Walk 9km every day before 9am	Daily
	Walk a marathon distance non-stop	1 Year
Mental Well-being	Meditate for 15 minutes a day	Daily
Academic	Study for a diploma in coaching and join a coaching industry body	1 Year
	Write a book on my alcohol-free journey	1 Year
	Read a wide range of philosophy and psychology books	5 Years
Adventure	Drive around the UK coastline doing 60 x 9km walks over a 4-month period	2 Years
Creative Challenges	Learn to play the piano to a good standard	2 Years
	Take an advanced guitar course	1 Year
Relationships	Do a hobby with my wife – walking	Daily
	Spend more time with my (grown up) children	Weekly
	Spend more time with my mother finding out more about her life	Daily
Gratitude	Do at least one good deed for another person every day	Daily

WHAT I LEARNT

IT'S THE JOURNEY NOT THE DESTINATION

One thing I learnt really early on, and I think was critical to my success in stopping drinking, was that the goal was the journey, not the destination. By this, I mean I was living it straight away. This does not apply to all goals because some are time-dependent, like, I'm going to stop drinking for 28 Days, 90 Days and 365 Days. But with a lot of goals, you can take out the time element and achieve them immediately.

I started to think of my goals in a different way. I was not thinking of them in finite, line-in-the-sand terms such as, I want to be five stone lighter, I want to have a 34-inch waist, or I want to have better skin. I wanted these things, of course, but these would be a 'give me' if I could set a goal that would put me on a trajectory to achieving them. By Month Five of stopping drinking alcohol, these had evolved into:

Journey Goal 1 – Every day, do not drink alcohol today

Journey Goal 2 – Every day, get up between 5am and 5.30am and go for a minimum 9km walk

Journey Goal 3 – Every day, meditate for 15 minutes

Of course, there were other smaller goals, but I knew that by achieving these three Journey Goals daily, I would put myself on the best trajectory to achieve ALL my goals and whys.

And guess what – it works. After nine months of following these Journey Goals, I was called in for my five-year NHS Health Check. The results showed that I had lost three stone in weight; my blood pressure was 115/80; my cholesterol was 3.49; and my overall risk of cardiovascular disease in the next 10 years was 5.1%. These were all achieved through Journey Goals.

I think that if I'd set the goal of 'I want to lose three stone in four months', it would have been an arduous journey. I'd have been weighing myself daily to see how much closer I was getting to the goal and constantly thinking about it, no doubt leading to some form of anxiety. Compare that to the Journey Goals, two of which are achieved by 9am every day, and it's a no-brainer.

The Journey Goals I was achieving daily had become my new habits. Without realising it, I had moved my body clock back three hours. To the rest of the world, I was getting up at some ridiculous hour, but to me 5am was the new 8am. I was walking at least nine kilometres, meditating on the walk, and planning my day. I showered, ate breakfast and was in the office by 9am, 9.30am at the latest. I was fitter; I could think quicker; I was more productive; I had my mojo back. This was the new me. It was how I now lived my life. I felt great. I was not on a treadmill of trying to achieve difficult goals and failing. I had made 'the journey the goal' and the targets were all falling into place.

In the book *Atomic Habits*, James Clear talks about success as not being once-in-a-lifetime transformations but a product of your daily habits. This is exactly what happened to me. He says, 'You should be far more concerned with your current trajectory than with your current results.'

GOAL SETTING TO THE NOW

I listened to an interview with *Lululemon* founder Chip Wilson on the Tim Ferris podcast in early 2021, where he said: 'When setting goals, set them in date order, with the furthest away first and work back to today, or now goals'.

In short, it's easier to set goals for today if you have goals for the week. It's easier to set goals for the week, if you have goals for the month. It's easier to set goals for the month, if you have goals for the year. It's easier to set a one-year goal if you have a five-year goal, and so on. So, if my one-year goal was to have spent the last year alcohol-free, the setting of daily Journey Goals was easy. Journey Goal 1 – every day, do not drink alcohol today.

If your goal is a someday goal, you should start at the top and work back. If it's a one-year goal, start there and work back. You want to take your goal and work back until you have your today goal.

SOMEDAY GOAL	What's the one thing I want to do someday?
FIVE-YEAR GOAL	Based on my someday goal, what's the one thing I can do in the next five years?
ONE-YEAR GOAL	Based on my five-year goal, what's the one thing I can do this year?
MONTHLY GOAL	Based on my one-year goal, what's the one thing I can do this month?
WEEKLY GOAL	Based on my one-month goal, what's the one thing I can do this week?
DAILY GOAL	Based on my one-week goal, what's the one thing I can do today?
RIGHT NOW GOAL	Based on my daily (today) goal, what's the one thing I can do right now?

If we take as an example my writing this book. A year ago, my goal setting and timing around the book would have been as follows:

One year – publish the book

Nine months – complete writing of manuscript for editing and production

Six months – complete 50% of writing of manuscript

One month – have structure and content planned

One week – plan outline content

Today – research alcohol-free book sector

LANDING THE PLANE – PRIORITISING GOALS

It's easy to get caught in the trap of having too many goals. How do you prioritise? Chris Wilson, founder of *Simplify Your Why*, says: 'If you have more than three priorities, you don't have priorities'. I love this line. It's so simple but so true. I now live by this.

In his book, *The 4 Disciplines of Execution*, Jim Huling uses the metaphor for goal selection of likening yourself to an air traffic controller, in charge of hundreds of circling aircraft. You decide which ones to land. The circling planes are your goals. There's only room to land one at a time. But how do you select the one to bring down to earth? Which one goal do you focus on? The big question you need to ask is: which goal, when achieved, will create the biggest impact on me and others around me?

Put these goals, or aircraft, onto a shortlist. Once you have chosen the goal to focus on, work out how you can objectively measure it and how you can achieve it. Take full ownership of it. Find one or two things that can help you achieve it. Keep a compelling scoreboard, as the way you keep score is a driver and should make you play the game to win.

Without a doubt, my aircraft was stopping drinking. I decided to land that plane. I could measure it very simply by saying each day, 'Today I will not drink'. I also put a 365-day calendar on my fridge door (the gateway to wine and beer). Each morning, I ticked off the previous day from the 28, 90 and 365-Day Challenges. This served as a constant reminder of how well I was doing. It became a ritual and a reinforcer of the success of my journey.

STEPS YOU CAN TAKE

STEP 1 – LONG-TERM & SHORT-TERM GOALS

Write down your 'whys' or goals for wanting to stop drinking alcohol. Then, split these into short-term and long-term goals.

STEP 2 – GOAL SETTING TO THE NOW

Complete the following...

SOMEDAY GOAL	What's the one thing you want to do someday?
FIVE-YEAR GOAL	Based on your someday goal, what's the one thing you can do in the next five years?
ONE-YEAR GOAL	Based on your five-year goal, what's the one thing you can do this year?
MONTHLY GOAL	Based on your one-year goal, what's the one thing you can do this month?
WEEKLY GOAL	Based on your one-month goal, what's the one thing you can do this week?
DAILY GOAL	Based on your one-week goal, what's the one thing you can do today?
RIGHT NOW GOAL	Based on your daily (today) goal, what's the one thing you can do right now?

STEP 3 – JOURNEY GOALS

Write down three things that you can do every day or regularly that will help you work towards achieving all your goals.

KEY LEARNINGS

- Get WISE about your WHYS!

- Set goals! Imagine asking the captain of a ship, 'Where are you heading?' and they say, 'I don't know.'

- Make the journey the goal and the targets are more likely to fall into place.

- Turn your goals into projects. With a project, you are always learning and growing. You can't fail a project because it's ongoing.

- 'If you have more than three priorities you don't have priorities'. Chris Wilson.

- It's easier to set goals for today if you have goals for the week. It's easier to set goals for the week if you have goals for the month, and so on.

- Make sure your daily goals put you on the best trajectory to achieving ALL of your goals.

- Stopping drinking is about changing your beliefs. By learning to believe in yourself, you can achieve anything you want through a few simple changes. The answers are already in your mind. You just need to discover where to find them.

CHAPTER 9
IDENTIFY YOUR VALUES

Setting goals and following your dreams becomes a lot easier once you have identified your true values and cemented your beliefs. By doing this, you will be better placed to find your purpose. Using these three proactive measures, you can create a mindset that will lead to a fulfilling life of fun and happiness.

Values are the universal concepts that unite people. They include concepts like fairness, justice, freedom and equality. Tony Robbins says they 'are like a compass that directs your life'. They motivate us, demotivate us and justify our behaviour.

MY STORY

This chapter focuses on my values, explains the process I followed to identify them, and offers you the opportunity to do the same.

I would like to stress at the outset that this chapter offers a structural process to identify your values. It is not meant to be rigid. It is simply a guide to help you find the values that define you.

I was starting to realise that to change my story I first needed to work out what my current story is and use this as the basis for creating the new one – the new me!

The alternative approach, which I was pretty much following, was not giving much thought to what my values, beliefs and purpose are, and leaving many things to chance. Just a few unhelpful values and a few hand-me-down beliefs can set up a world full of anxiety, stress, pain and unhappiness.

When I started the process of reviewing, deleting and inserting new values, I realised I was living in my own self-made cycle of get up, go to work, watch TV, drink wine, go to bed, get up and do it again.

Don't get me wrong – I have always enjoyed my life. I love running my own business and I have a wide range of hobbies and a beautiful family. But something was wrong. I was drinking too much to really appreciate what I had.

MY VALUES LIST

I'd never sat down before with pen and paper or keyboard and screen and thought about listing my values. But it is probably one of the best things I have ever done. It's the start of the process of working out what it is you stand for, what you'd like to stand for and what you don't want to stand for.

The science says that values motivate actions and help us make decisions. For example, if one of my main values is to live a healthy life, then I will start seeing the world through this value and will be more likely to participate in healthy activities as opposed to unhealthy pursuits. It's obvious really, but it is such an eye-opener to write it down.

If you asked most people what their values are, they'd probably feel uncomfortable with the question because many of us just do not have time to think about it and don't know the answers off the top of our heads.

I made two lists:

MY POSITIVE VALUES
- health
- family
- learning/wisdom
- love
- creativity
- gratitude
- success
- humour
- fun
- courage
- fairness
- temperance

MY NEGATIVE VALUES
- anger
- conflict
- failure
- not believing in myself
- bad temper
- unhealthy lifestyle

I then slept on this.

Not putting my health and fitness first had been my major problem. I realised that I needed to be fit, healthy and calm in order to give my best to others.

I knew I wanted to be: caring, successful, hardworking, family-orientated and remain happily-married.

I knew I loved learning and I wanted to give back. I wanted to continue to be a good father, husband, son, brother and friend.

By being alcohol-free, I wanted to help others. I wanted to be an author writing about healthy living, and an alcohol-free living coach helping others along their pathways to AF freedom.

I realised the core values I now live by, and will never stray from, are:

love, family, connection, fun, humour, meaning, happiness, caring, calmness, creativity, physical and mental health, learning and wisdom, giving back, gratitude, doing things right now, courage, fairness and valuing relationships above all material things.

WHAT I LEARNT

THE MAP IS NOT THE TERRITORY

One of the most exciting discoveries I made is that I can reorganise my values. I can add, delete and restructure them to support the life I want.

The science says that all information must enter through our minds. The brain uses our values and beliefs as a filter system to influence how we perceive the world around us.

Neuro Linguistic Programming, or NLP, sees values as those things that provide direction in our lives. We move towards things we value and away from things we don't. We pay attention to those things that we feel are important and ignore those things we don't.

NLP suggests that everyone looks at the world, or the territory, through their own map – a map built on their values and beliefs. A map unique to them. No two maps are the same.

Our lives are so full of information that unless we're selective, we will quickly be overwhelmed. To prevent this overload, we tend to pay most attention to the things we value and ignore the rest. For this reason, each and every one of us has a unique model of reality. Our worlds are all different because we pay most attention to those things that align with our values.

For example, someone with a map that is made up of values and beliefs including 'drinking alcohol is a fun way to relax and makes them happy' might look at a glass of wine, the territory, as something that will take all their problems away. Another person's map comprising values and beliefs that 'alcohol consumption is unhealthy and can lead to major health problems', will look at the same glass of wine in a very different way.

This is really powerful stuff and is at the heart of the secret to stopping drinking and going alcohol-free. By changing your values and beliefs you can change your story, your world and the direction of your life.

EMBRACE YOUR VALUES

Create new pathways in your mind by reminding yourself of your values and their order of importance over and over again. As Henry David Thoreau tells us, 'As a single footstep will not make a path on the earth, so a single thought will not make a pathway in the mind.' This is supported by the Buddhist teaching that, 'Whatever we think about regularly becomes the inclination of our mind.'

The *One Year No Beer Challenge* tells you to bring your values to life, bring them into your world, to push this information down into the very core of your being, to be stored in your subconscious so that you automatically live by these ideals.

I then did three things that worked for me:

1. Create a life force 'Who am I?' statement. Mine is: 'I am a sober, healthy, fun-loving, creative, family man'. Put the life-force statement somewhere you can see it on a daily basis, maybe next to the bathroom mirror! Or,

as this is just one sentence, perhaps learn it by heart and repeat it to yourself in front of the mirror each morning. One of the keys to happiness for me is to live by this statement every single day.

2. Put your values list somewhere visible so you can read over them every single day until you absorb their guidance.

3. Continually ask yourself what someone would do or how someone would react, who valued 'health' as one of their top values. Or if 'fun' is your number one value then how would this make you feel about your up-and-coming activity?

This trains your mind to recognise these values as core ideals to live by. Your values will then program your subconscious mind by creating new pathways to accept these ideas and protect them by making sure you adhere to these values.

Once the powerful primitive part of your brain supports these ideas, your world will be transformed.

VALUES & RULES

Once you have your list of values, it is critical to create a rule system around them because living by your values is totally dependent on these rules. The key is not whether your rules are right or wrong but whether they empower or disempower you.

Here is an example of my main values and the rules I linked to each:

VALUE	RULE
Health	Walk 9km a day
	Don't drink alcohol
Mental health	Meditate daily
Meaning	Read philosophy daily

Love & family	It's hard to make rules around this because it is not a 'to do' list. I just became more loving and wanted to express this. This manifests itself in things like saying 'I love you' to my wife and hugging my children more often
Learning	Listen to a podcast at least twice a week
	Always have a book that I am currently reading
	Learn a new song on the piano and/or guitar every week
Giving back	Do a charitable thing each day
Gratefulness	Write down three things I am grateful for every day
Fun	Smile as much as I can
Connection	Meet one new person each day

STEPS YOU CAN TAKE

STEP 1 - POSITIVE & NEGATIVE VALUES

Make a list of your positive and negative values.

POSITIVE VALUES	NEGATIVE VALUES
Here is a list of positive values to choose from. This is by no means exhaustive, but it's a good start: achievement, balance, compassion, determination, fairness, fun, gratitude, happiness, humility, influence, justice, kindness, leadership, optimism, peace, respect, spirituality, teamwork, understanding, wealth, wisdom, zest.	Here's a few I'd like to avoid. Again, this is in no way exhaustive: anger, bad temper, conflict, discouragement, disinterest, envy, failure, forgetting your worth, guilt, giving up easily, jealousy, not believing in yourself, not standing up for yourself, overthinking, trying to please everyone.

The idea isn't to pick solely from the list, but to expand the list and add your own values based on your own experiences and personality.

STEP 2 – REVIEW & FINALISE YOUR LIST

Sleep on your first list and add to it by identifying the core values that support the vision you have of yourself. These values are the ones you want to live your life by and never stray from.

STEP 3 – LOOK AFTER YOUR LIST

Keep it somewhere safe so you can refer back to it.

Review regularly. Your vision of yourself will evolve over time, so your values need to evolve with this vision.

KEY LEARNINGS

- Setting goals and following your dreams becomes a lot easier once you have identified your true values and cemented your beliefs.

- Values are the universal concepts that unite people. They include concepts like fairness, justice, freedom and equality.

- Values motivate us, demotivate us and justify our behaviour.

- You can add, delete and restructure your values to support the life you want.

- All information has to enter through our minds and the brain uses our values and beliefs as a filter system to influence how we perceive the world around us.

- Everyone looks at the world, or the territory, through their own map, a map built on their values and beliefs. A map unique to them. No two maps are the same.

- By changing your values and beliefs you can change your story, your world and the direction of your life.

- Embrace your values. Put your values list somewhere visible so you can read over them every single day until you absorb their guidance.

- Create a rule system around your values to empower you.

CHAPTER 10
THERE'S NOTHING YOU CAN'T DO - CEMENT YOUR BELIEFS

Beliefs are wide and varied and range from what we believe about the creation of the universe to what we choose to eat and drink! They are a major part of defining who we are. We are not our behaviour; we are our beliefs.

MY STORY

In the first few weeks of alcohol-free living, I took a long, hard look at my beliefs.

I realised that my beliefs are simply assumptions which I hold to be true and which may – or may not be – based on facts.

One of the first major changes I made to my belief system, was to make THERE IS NOTHING I CAN'T DO a central part of who I am.

I had left my beliefs unchecked and ended up with a whole host of limiting, unhelpful beliefs that I either inherited or picked up from family, government, colleagues and the world around me.

The list of beliefs is potentially endless. So it was important I focused in on the ones that are central to what makes me me. I also tried to remember where these beliefs had come from.

Rather than list all my beliefs, which would take a very long time, I concentrated on those that are relevant to pursuing a healthy, alcohol-free life.

These are the beliefs I had at the very start of my alcohol-free journey, in no particular order. What is interesting is that all the negative beliefs I identified with, came from me. If they came from me, I thought, I could easily get rid of them.

POSITIVE BELIEF	WHERE IT CAME FROM
I am intelligent	Passing exams, graduating, life experience
I am optimistic	Childhood – mother
I am reliable	Being a dad, running my own company
I like to win	Childhood – my older brother
I am kind/I am a good father, son, husband	Helping others – my wife, children, mother
I am forgiving	School, mother, church
I am loving	Mother
I am ambitious	Childhood
I am loyal	Parents
I am honest	Parents
I am courageous	Parents
I've worked hard for what I have	Parents
Luck is where opportunity meets hard work	Childhood
The world's your oyster	Mother

POSITIVE BELIEF	WHERE IT CAME FROM
If it does not kill you, it makes you stronger	Childhood
Question everything – don't take things at face value	Parents
I am always aware of my surroundings	Childhood
I am successful	Going to university, running my own business, being entrepreneurial
I am creative	My work and my hobbies – guitar, piano, painting, photography, writing
I am a marketing expert	My work
I am proud to be Welsh	Childhood
I love sport	Childhood, playing golf, being a children's football coach

NEGATIVE BELIEF	WHERE IT CAME FROM
I am fat	Me
I am unhealthy	Me
I cannot stop drinking for more than a week	Me
I am a loser because I cannot control my drinking habit long term – I don't think I can ever completely give up alcohol	Me
I lack self-discipline	Me
I am a drinker	Me
I am short-tempered	Me

NEW BELIEFS I WANTED

I had to get rid of the negative beliefs – they were holding me back. But I also needed to add some 'superpower' beliefs to the positive ones to 'supercharge' me, to create the new me. The big two super beliefs I chose are:

'There's Nothing I Can't Do' and **'I'll Always Find A Way That's Morally Right'**

I also added the following, which I told myself would become my new mantras:

I am sober

I can be fit and healthy

I want to be fit and healthy

I will be fit and healthy

I also added my achievements to my beliefs, because they reinforce them. I am an LSE graduate, which reinforces the belief that I am intelligent. An intelligent person would not choose to be unhealthy. An intelligent person would question, 'Is alcohol good for my health?'

This new 'I am' that I was developing – my values, my beliefs and my purpose – would become my new identity.

WHAT I LEARNT

LIMITING BELIEFS & ELEPHANTS

When circus elephants are young, their trainers tie a rope to their back leg and wrap it around a stake in the ground. The baby elephant is not strong enough to break free and hurts its leg in trying to do so. In time, it learns to be constrained and gives up trying to escape.

Later, as a fully mature adult, the trainer only has to tie a small rope around the elephant's leg and attach the other end to any pole or stake, and a 5,000kg elephant believes it is trapped. Even though it has amazing strength and power to break free. It has been conditioned not to use its power and strength.

Many of us are like elephants – powerful spiritual beings, with amazing strength, yet due to conditioning we hold ourselves back and fail to realise our potential. We live out the same beliefs that we have been programmed to believe without ever questioning them.

Life is one gigantic self-fulfilling prophecy. We spend our whole life telling stories about ourselves. These stories become real and are often full of debilitating and limiting beliefs.

I was telling myself a story that I was a drinker. I needed to drink for my job. It made me relax. It made me happy.

EXAMPLES OF BELIEFS

Psychologists say that beliefs fall into two main types: *core beliefs* and *truth beliefs*.

Core beliefs are formed in childhood. They come from parents, friends, education or you could have worked them out yourself. Core beliefs are things like, 'family is more important than work'; 'drink-driving is wrong'; 'I would never be unfaithful'; 'murder is wrong'. These core beliefs are hard to change.

Truth beliefs come from lots of sources. We believe them to be true and they become part of us. They are part of our identity. The good thing about these types of belief is they can be changed more easily than core beliefs.

Beliefs live deep in our unconscious mind, a place not easily accessible and well-defended by our conscious mind. Throughout the journey, I told myself, and I believed it, that I am alcohol-free, and I can easily change my habits. I truly believe this!

Here's a generic – not my own – list of positive and negative beliefs:

POSITIVE BELIEFS	NEGATIVE BELIEFS
My family will always support me no matter what	Everyone knows I have zero willpower
I have the courage to bounce back	I can't compete with these guys
I can learn to change my habits	I don't believe I can do it
I deserve love	I'm not good enough
I am a good (loving) person	I don't deserve love
I am fine as I am	I am a bad person
I am happy	I am terrible
I am worthy	I am unhappy
I am worthwhile	I am worthless (inadequate)
I am honourable	I am not lovable
I am lovable	I deserve only bad things
I am deserving (fine/OK)	I am permanently damaged
I deserve good things	I am ugly (my body is hateful)
I am (can be) healthy	I am stupid (not smart enough)
I am fine (attractive/lovable)	I am insignificant (unimportant)
I am intelligent (able to learn)	
I am significant (important)	I am a disappointment
I deserve to live	I deserve to die
I deserve to be happy	I deserve to be miserable
I can be trusted	I am different (don't belong)
I can (learn to) trust myself	I cannot be trusted
I can trust my judgement	I cannot trust myself
I can choose who to trust	I cannot trust my judgment
I can (learn to) take care of myself	I cannot trust anyone
	I cannot protect myself
I can safely feel (show) my emotions	It's not OK to feel (show) my emotions
I can make my needs known	I cannot stand up for myself

POSITIVE BELIEFS	NEGATIVE BELIEFS
I can choose to let it out	I cannot let it out
I am now in control	I am not in control
I am strong	I am powerless (helpless)
I can get what I want	I am weak
I can succeed	I cannot get what I want
I can be myself (make mistakes)	I am a failure (will fail)
	I cannot succeed
I can handle it	I must be perfect (please everyone)
I am capable	
	I cannot stand it
	I am inadequate

BUILDING BELIEFS

The way to build beliefs is through small, daily actions. This creates reference points for you to gather evidence that this belief holds true.

Every day that you remain alcohol-free, you are building a firm belief that you can thrive without alcohol. You are taking apart those limiting beliefs around alcohol and building a new empowering belief that you no longer need it.

You can use this same understanding to build other healthy beliefs. I now have a belief that I am a person that exercises every day and I support this belief on a daily basis by walking 9KM BY 9AM. But this does not have to mean a very long walk or a massive gym session. You could include using the stairs at work.

The key is to complete some form of exercise every day, even if it is only for a few minutes. This will train you to believe that you are the sort of person that exercises every day. Once the belief grows, you can create a more adventurous exercise plan, safe in the knowledge that you will subconsciously want to do it because you believe that you're someone who exercises every day.

This is exactly what I did with 9KM BY 9AM. Science has also shown that missing the odd day does not materially affect habit formation. If you can imagine that each positive action casts a vote for this new belief and each time you don't exercise, it casts a vote against. As long as you receive enough votes for your new belief, it will stick.

Anthony Robbins suggests we build beliefs like we would a table. The belief starts out as the table top and we use references to create the legs. The stronger the references, the stronger the legs, which creates a solid belief. You can also apply this idea to breaking up limiting beliefs.

STEPS YOU CAN TAKE

STEP 1 – LIST YOUR BELIEFS

Note down as many of your personal beliefs as you can.

Then, take a step back and decide if these beliefs are helpful or not.

Group them into positive and negative beliefs.

Try and remember where these beliefs come from. Was it a hand-me-down from a parent or friend? Or was it an experience you had in the past?

STEP 2 – SHOULD THEY STAY OR SHOULD THEY GO?

Decide if you want to keep these beliefs or change them. This is how you 'weed the garden of your mind', as Andy Ramage says.

The aim is to highlight and support your positive beliefs, while undermining and breaking down any negative ones.

You can decide what to believe, and by doing so, influence the way you feel.

STEP 3 – CHALLENGE YOUR LIMITING BELIEFS

List the beliefs you have about yourself, which you think are limiting. Remember all beliefs can be challenged.

Take each limiting belief and ask the following questions. Let's use one of my old limiting beliefs, 'I like drinking alcohol', as an example:

- Does this belief improve your life?
- Is this belief good for your health?
- Does this belief have any harmful consequences for you or others?

KEY LEARNINGS

- Beliefs are assumptions that you hold to be true and may, or may not, be based on facts.
- Beliefs are part of our identity.
- We can consciously decide what we believe in – and what we don't.
- Your story starts with who you are. By changing your beliefs, you can change your story and that will change your life.
- Some beliefs are limiting and debilitating.
- Many of us live out the same beliefs that we have been programmed to believe without ever questioning them.
- Beliefs can be changed.
- Focus on what you want – see it as real. I am a non-drinker, I am healthy, I meditate, there is nothing I cannot do. If you start doing this, your identity shifts and you become it.
- 'We are what we repeatedly do. Excellence is not an act but a habit'. Aristotle

CHAPTER 11
FIND YOUR PURPOSE

Your purpose is a core part of your identity. It embodies your values and your beliefs. It is your mission in life.

MY STORY

I love these words by Mary Oliver, from The Summer Day:
Tell me, what is it you plan to do
With your one wild and precious life?

My purpose is more of a eulogy than a resumé.

I used this approach as a great way to focus in on my purpose, simply because what is written on a gravestone tends to be how others remember that person.

'He was a great friend. He made changes in his own life that inspired me to make changes. He was there for me.' Wow! That sounds a lot better than, 'He worked in marketing for 40 years.'

This eulogy approach tells us more about a person. It reveals more about the true self.

When I first started the journey, I wrote down what I believed to be my old story and the new story I wanted to be.

My old story was, 'I was someone who from the outside looked successful, with both material and social wealth, nice house, sports car, lovely family, own business. But I had fallen into the trap of drinking most days to relax and escape from the stresses of the world. This was making me very unfit; it was eating away at my relationships; it had made me anxious, overweight and irritable. I was holding myself back from being the real me.' When I read this now, after more than a year of being alcohol-free, it does not sound good. I think to myself – what an idiot! Why did I not do something about it earlier?

My new story is 'I control alcohol. It does not control me. I am healthy and fit. I am a better if not the best husband, dad, son. I plan to learn new things every day and evolve my business.'

When I was growing up in the 1970s and 1980s, if you were the son of a doctor, there was a good chance you'd end up becoming a doctor. Not much has changed in this respect. If you were the son of an F1 world champion, there was a good chance you would be a successful racing driver. Look at Damon and Graham Hill, Nico and Keke Rosberg, Mick and Michael Schumacher.

Part of my purpose came from my parents, but it was not their jobs that I wanted to follow. My dad had been in the Royal Navy in the Second World War and had travelled around the world. I believe his stories of travelling to places such as India and Singapore gave me the appetite to travel. Part of my purpose as a younger man was to travel. I wanted to leave Cardiff. I wanted to explore the world.

My mother is very stoic. She always worked hard, putting her family first and made sure we were always fed and clothed and loved. She is always smiling and happy. My optimistic outlook on life and putting my family first definitely comes from her influence on me.

When I was in my 20s, my purpose was to travel, see the world, have fun, learn, be successful and always give my best. I think I arrived at this purpose sometime around my early 20s. I think very few young people know their purpose until around this age as they are still being formed. Looking back, I spent my 20s and 30s working out what I would really like to do with my life.

By the time I hit my 30s, I had travelled to over 50 countries, and lived and worked as an expat in Singapore. I met my wife there and by my early 30s, we were both back in the UK, living in a lovely London commuter village and raising a young family. I left the world of being an employee and set up my own company. I had found my purpose. I was happy. Very simply, I was caring for my beautiful family.

My purpose today, and for the foreseeable future, is still to care for my family but also to help others.

Going through this life-changing experience of stopping drinking, I have discovered who I am. I have taken away the shadow that alcohol cast on my thoughts about myself, about others and about my relationships. I want to help change the way people think about alcohol, about their purpose and about their mental health. The first step along this new purpose path of mine is writing this book and becoming an alcohol-free life coach.

FINDING MY PURPOSE

After identifying my values and cementing my beliefs, I looked at what drives me, what I was good at, and what I would like to do with my life. What I wrote in my journal was as follows:

Things that drive me: getting fitter – through walking; my family – spending time with my wife, children, mother; learning new things every day – reading philosophy, science, history.

Things I think I am good at: writing; playing the guitar and piano; photography; making videos – in front and behind camera; talking!

What I would like to do with the rest of my life: be remembered by people who have met me as someone who cared about them; help people see how to change their relationship with alcohol.

My draft purpose statement: 'I am a healthy, sober, family man who loves learning about life, arts, culture and helping people find well-being.'

WHAT I LEARNT

WHAT IS PURPOSE AND WHY IS IT SO IMPORTANT?

Your goals will be easier to achieve if they are in line with your purpose. Your purpose can change over time just like your values and beliefs can evolve. My purpose when I was in my 20s is different to what it is today.

Everybody has a purpose. We can't all be Paul McCartney; we can't all be Oprah Winfrey – but we do all have a purpose, a mission. Your mission or your purpose doesn't have to be great or grandiose. It could be, 'I want to make things with my hands and love my family'. You don't have to be Greta Thunberg and change the world. The main thing is that you're happy with your purpose.

If you feel contentment, then you are pursuing your purpose.

DON'T FIGHT THE WIND

I heard a podcast interview with actor Rainn Wilson and scholar Reza Aslan, who talked about purpose being like a sailboat journey. I thought this was a beautiful way to explain it and it went something like this:

Think of your purpose as a life journey on a sailboat to an island. You are at the helm, steering the boat through the waters of your day-to-day life to follow your purpose. There are forces at play that are not within your control, like the winds and storms. But there are others that you can control, such as learning to use the sails and rudder to stay on course and ride out storms that try their best to blow you off your course.

Sometimes you can't sail the direct course - you must follow the wind. Sometimes there will be no wind and you need to use other sources, like rowing or using a motor. But it is the bigger force of whatever we call God, the spiritual force, the godly force around you that will keep you moving throughout life to your destination.

If you're fighting the wind, you're not pursuing your purpose. You know when you're moving smoothly through life, smoothly over the water, that you're doing things right. You are in line with the island that you're heading to: you are in line with your purpose.

IT'S NOT YOUR JOB

Reza Aslan also says, 'Have a mission not a job. Your mission is bigger than the things that you do'. Your purpose is not your job, it's your mission. A doctor's purpose, for example, is not to be a doctor, but to help others. A mission is much wider than a job. If your purpose is to help others you could be a doctor, you could be a charity worker, you could care for people.

WHERE DOES PURPOSE COME FROM?

Your purpose naturally flows from your values. If you see yourself as a caring person, then part of your purpose may well be to help others. If you see yourself as a creative person, then your purpose could be to write, to make furniture or to paint.

Purpose tends to come from your parents, older siblings, relatives, friends or teachers. It can also come from your life experiences and the things that resonate with you.

FACING YOUR FEARS HELPS

When drafting, developing and deciding on your purpose, never be afraid. Never fear that you may not be able to follow the purpose you decide you want to follow.

The adage is, 'You need to step up to the line, be counted, be the man'. However, I think Joseph Campbell puts it more eloquently. He said, 'The cave you fear to enter holds the treasure you seek.'

Once you face your fears, they lose their power – when you face them head-on you are dealing with them. Once you have the awareness of the 'monster', you can start dealing with the 'monster' because you can see it for what it really is. This is exactly what happened to me after I stopped drinking alcohol. All the fears of failing disappeared as soon as I started to see the 'monster', in my case alcohol, for what it really was – poison.

The Tibetan Buddhist teacher Pema Chödrön says, 'Only to the extent that we expose ourselves over and over again to annihilation can that which is indestructible be found in us.' I took this to mean that I had had it with drinking. 35 years was more than enough. Thousands of hangovers, hundreds of thousands of anxious thoughts. It had not killed me, but it had made me stronger. I used this strength to keep going and finally put all my fears about it to death.

Chödrön says that fear is a natural reaction to moving closer to the truth. If we commit ourselves to staying right where we are, then our experience becomes very vivid. Things become very clear when there is nowhere to escape to. This clarity is a matter of becoming intimate with fear and, rather than treating it as a problem to be solved, using it as a tool with which to dismantle all our familiar structures of being, 'a complete undoing of old ways of seeing, hearing, smelling, tasting, and thinking.' Bravery is not the absence of fear but the intimacy with fear.

This wonderful alcohol-free living experience has made me realise that true happiness and contentment are already here. I just did not know where to look. I am not escaping any more. I love my life. I love my purpose and I have no desire to escape this alcohol-free world.

PURPOSE CHANGES OVER TIME

Like beliefs, purpose changes over time. My purpose when I was a young man in my teens and 20s, is very different to what it is today. My purpose has included exploring the world, helping others, learning new things every day, and helping change the way people think about alcohol and their mental health.

If you are the same person you were one year ago, five years ago, ten years ago, then you've not challenged your values. You are not challenging what you are doing. I'm definitely a different person. If I had not challenged my values, I almost definitely would still be drinking, and I would not have this new purpose.

PURPOSE DEPENDS ON LIFE CIRCUMSTANCES

Abraham Maslow's famous paper, *A Theory of Human Motivation*, states that people are motivated to fulfil basic needs before moving on to other, more advanced, needs. Maslow believed that people have an inborn desire to be self-actualised, that is, 'to be all they can be'. In order to achieve these ultimate goals, however, several more basic needs must be met, such as the need for food, safety, love, and self-esteem.

This means your purpose will have a different meaning depending on your life circumstances. If you do not have a roof over your head, your purpose becomes to survive. This can be seen in 2020 when a lot of people's purpose became to survive COVID-19.

ENTHUSIASM

Remember nothing is ever achieved without enthusiasm. I've only been able to get up every morning at 5am and walk 9KM BY 9AM because I want to. This goal fits with my purpose.

I'll end what I learnt with a great line from Rainn Wilson who says, 'Your purpose is to find your purpose'.

STEPS YOU CAN TAKE

If you don't know your purpose, it does not mean you don't have one. It just means you have not found it yet.

The following steps will help you create a draft purpose statement:

STEP 1 – WHAT DRIVES YOU?

What are the things that drive you? Make a list.

STEP 2 – WHAT ARE YOU GOOD AT?

List the things you are good at.

STEP 3 – WHAT WOULD YOU LIKE TO DO WITH THE REST OF YOUR LIFE?

Make a list of the things you would really like to do.

STEP 4 – STATEMENT

Write your draft Purpose Statement based on the answers to Steps 1, 2 and 3. Here is mine again: 'I am a healthy, sober, family man who loves learning about life, arts, culture and helping people find well-being.'

KEY LEARNINGS

- Your purpose is a core part of your identity. It embodies your values and your beliefs. It is your mission in life.

- By identifying your true values and beliefs, you will cement your purpose to support the life you desire and ultimately bring you more happiness.

- Setting goals and following your dreams becomes a lot easier if you have worked out what your purpose is.

- Everybody has a purpose. Your purpose is to find a purpose.

- If you don't know your purpose, then you have not found it yet.
- What you want written on your gravestone – that's your purpose.
- Your purpose is not your job, it's your mission.
- Purpose changes over time.
- If you feel contentment, then you are pursuing your purpose.

CHAPTER 12
CHANGING YOUR BELIEFS ABOUT ALCOHOL

Former US marine, consciousness expert and black belt in jujitsu, Rabbi Mordecai Finley talks about levels of deepness in the mind using a martial arts belt metaphor. He says that starting to understand how your mind works gets you a yellow belt. Understanding the issues you have and how to retrain your brain to think how you want it to think, takes you to a blue belt. But you could go further and go for a black belt, allowing you to dig really deep.

MY STORY

From day one, I wanted to dig deep. I wanted to understand how I could influence my unconscious mind, the place where all my beliefs are stored.

I earned my blue belt and created new pathways and new ways of thinking. I am now working towards my black belt.

I learnt that to change my life, it is critical to change my story. To do this, I needed to change my beliefs. But how could I do this?

My main limiting belief, without one shadow of doubt, was that I was NOT 100% in control of my alcohol intake.

I had some control but I could not stop drinking for more than a few days at a time. I drank most evenings and every weekend. I was overweight, unfit and short of breath, all caused by this one belief that I could not control alcohol. So, it controlled me.

I asked myself this question: 'Would I run my computer on 35-year-old-software?' Of course not.

I pulled out the old CD with my limiting beliefs on and scratched it so it will never play again, even if I ever try to reinsert it.

My identity is defined by who I believe I am and who I believe I am not!

My decisions are controlled by my identity.

My best thinking had got me where I was. The big question was, could I be somewhere better? Yes, I could.

I realised the secret is to understand that beliefs are not always facts! Just because I think it, doesn't make it true!

I took away the power of all the limiting beliefs I had about alcohol that were holding me back. I wrote down: 'I cannot have fun without alcohol', 'Alcohol relaxes me', and others, on Post-it notes and put them on my computer screen so I could see them throughout the day. I continually challenged them. I began to realise they were all simply not true.

I now think of limiting beliefs as ice cubes in a heated swimming pool of beliefs. Very quickly they melt.

ONE YEAR FROM NOW

At the start of my alcohol-free journey, I pretended that in one year's time, I would have just lived the greatest year of my life.

I am healthier and fitter than I have been since my 20s. This has been the best year of my life so far because I have got myself back. I have loving relationships with my wife, my children and my family.

Every day of that year I told myself – alcohol is no longer important to me. I could take it or leave it and I decided to leave it.

OLD & NEW IDENTITY

I also wrote down my old identity and the new identity I wanted. Here are some of the items in my lists:

OLD TRAITS/ VALUES TO BANISH FROM MY ID	TRAITS I WANTED TO KEEP/AM PROUD OF	NEW TRAITS/ VALUES TO BUILD ON/ADD TO MY ID
I am a drinker/ boozer	I am successful	I am sober
I am short tempered	I am an entrepreneur	I am fit
I am angry	I am an expert in marketing/PR/ sponsorship	I am healthy
I am fat/ overweight	I am creative	I am a great dad
I am unhealthy	I am Welsh	I am a great husband
I am unfit	I am from Cardiff	I am caring
	I am an LSE graduate	I am compassionate
	I am a good father, husband, son, brother, friend	I am present
		I am grateful
		I am unstoppable

I had created a compelling future for myself. Every day, I told myself who I am through incantations. 'I am a non-drinker; I am healthy'. This reinforced my new story. Compelling future statements can be incredibly powerful. Just look at what President John F Kennedy told the American people in 1960. He said the USA would put a man on the moon by the end of that decade. That was a compelling future. And they did it.

I had to see everything as real: 'I am sober'; 'I am a great dad'. This is how I shifted my identity.

To make a shift in my identity I needed to redefine myself. I am not my behaviour – I am my beliefs. This one saying is so powerful because if you just stop drinking using only the willpower method, you really are still a drinker. It is only when you firmly believe you are a non-drinker that you free yourself.

CHANGE YOUR STORY, CHANGE YOUR LIFE

I had to relabel myself. I had to get rid of those old Post-it notes that were stuck on me. I was not dependent on alcohol. I did not need alcohol to be successful in my job entertaining my clients. I did not need alcohol to relax. I did not need alcohol to have fun.

I had to create new pathways in my mind. A branch of psychology called neuroplasticity helped me do this; to see alcohol for what it really is.

A quote written over 170 years ago by US philosopher Henry David Thoreau was at the heart of my success. This is the quote I put at the very start of the book, and I will be forever grateful to him for writing it. He said, 'As a single footstep will not make a path on the earth, so a single thought will not make a pathway in the mind. To make a deep physical path, we walk again and again. To make a deep mental path, we must think over and over the kind of thoughts we wish to dominate our lives.' This is supported by the Buddhist teaching: 'Whatever you think about regularly becomes the inclination of your mind.' This is the basis of what is today called neuroplasticity.

To make a pathway in the forest, we walk again and again. Similarly, to make a deep mental path, we must think again and again the thoughts that we want to dominate our lives. I told myself many times each day that I was a non-drinker and supported it with hard evidence on how bad alcohol was for my well-being. I made alcohol the enemy. I saw if for what it really was – poison.

In the early days of going AF, I had to fight myself, my ego. I had to un-brainwash myself. For 35 years, I had sung the same song.

The way I successfully changed my belief about alcohol was to wage a war on my belief that alcohol was part of my life; it was too hard to live my life and be happy without it. I would be boring if I did not drink. I would be an outcast – a social pariah.

THE TIPPING POINT

The Tipping Point, the moment when I first realised that I truly believed alcohol is bad for me, came in the third week after I stopped drinking.

Over the first three weeks, I submerged myself in Quit Lit, (short for Quit Literature or alcohol-free living books), podcasts, YouTube videos, websites, and social media alcohol-free groups. It was like fighting an inner war against the control over my alcohol consumption – my alcohol habit.

This Quit Lit helped me build the case against alcohol. The more information I sourced, the closer I moved towards the Tipping Point, the point of no return, the point where it was no longer possible to say, 'Alcohol relaxes me'; 'Alcohol is fun'; 'Alcohol gives me confidence'.

I could feel this Tipping Point getting closer and closer. It was exciting. It was like I was 3-0 down at half time in a football match. To many, that would be game over, but I knew I could turn things around. I had a plan which was getting stronger by the day, fuelled through the Quit Lit. The second half (of my life) had begun.

With every book, every podcast, every video I consumed, I was coming back into the game and scoring goals. It really was a game of two halves. I always knew alcohol was bad for me; I now believed it.

It was like a new voice had emerged inside me, a new part to my ego, and I really wanted it to grow and grow. By wanting this so much, it was starting to happen.

Looking back now, over a year after stopping, I have realised that the inner war is at its bloodiest in the early days, when the ego is fighting hard to hang onto the old beliefs and using everything possible to try to win, including mental and physical cravings. In the first week, these happened almost every minute as it is all I thought about. But as the days went by and I took more information on board, the cravings became fewer and the whole process became easier and easier.

WHAT I LEARNT

WHAT IS EGO?

There are many definitions of ego, but for the purposes of this book I'm going to define it simply as the voice that tells you what to do. It is your inner narrator and your sense of yourself.

It's critical to get an understanding of what it is because once you know your enemies, it's easier to hatch the plan to beat them.

According to Dan Harris in his book *10% Happier*, your ego comments on your actions and behaviour from the moment you open your eyes in the morning until you drift off to sleep at night, telling you what to do and what not to do.

If you believe deep down that alcohol is good for you, then your ego will support that belief. It's the voice that says: 'Go on! Have a drink, you deserve it! It's been a long hard day!'

The ego and alcohol are not the best mix and can lead very quickly to anxious thoughts - quite the opposite of relaxing.

The ego is obsessed with the past and the future and through this obsession, neglects the present, keeping you from fully living there. The ego loves to dwell in the past and thrives on drama by keeping old wounds open. It's the reason people bear grudges and can't let petty things go and move on. Sound familiar?

It is never satisfied. It will never be content and will never be perfectly happy.

The ego constantly assesses your worth against the appearance, wealth and social status of others, but will always find you failing. No matter how smart, beautiful or wealthy you may be, according to your ego, there's always someone smarter, more beautiful or wealthier.

So that's what you're up against! How the hell do you control it?

CONTROLLING YOUR EGO

The way I controlled my ego is through the skill of mindfulness.

To truly understand yourself and the beliefs you hold, you need to step outside yourself and observe who you are. A great way to do this is through meditation.

Through meditation, you can find spaces between the hundreds of thousands of thoughts that continually ring around your head. It is in these spaces that you can start to see what you believe and question whether those beliefs are right.

By doing this regularly you learn to control your thoughts, slow them down, dismiss them. This allows you to become calmer and nurtures your ability to build a time gap in how you react to events. The New You does not react to events. It responds to them, and this is a key difference.

For me, meditation and mindfulness are critical parts of the process to achieving behavioural changes - whether it's stopping drinking, changing your career, deciding to move house, deciding to do anything different.

MAKE IT RAIN

One of the foremost mindfulness and mediation experts in the world is Tara Brach. Through her guided meditations, I learnt how to dig deep into my mind and evaluate my beliefs.

Tara teaches the RAIN method – a series of four stages to accepting negative feelings or something you would like to overcome, whether it be anxiety, depression, guilt, death or, in this case, alcohol.

So, if my ego was telling me to drink alcohol because it was good and would relax me, I acknowledged this and accepted it. I did not deny it was not happening. I did not run away from it.

RAIN is an acronym:

Recognise that you think drinking alcohol is good for you. Then...

Allow this feeling/thought to exist. Next...

Investigate its effects and what it does to you. This is where you can feed in the new data from the Quit Lit. Finally...

Nurture the thoughts and start to separate yourself from this way of thinking through the practice of non-identification.

By non-identification, I told myself that the facts just don't add up. Alcohol can't be good for me. I'm only thinking this because I have been brainwashed. I am not stupid. I just need to ride it out and soon it will go away because I know the truth is that alcohol is bad for me.

By doing this, I was able to separate myself from my emotions and beliefs. I created new beliefs in my unconscious mind by repeatedly telling myself alcohol was bad for me, supported by facts and figures from the Quit Lit and, thereby, conquered my ego.

STEPS YOU CAN TAKE

STEP 1 – LIMITING BELIEFS

Write down on a sticky note all the beliefs you have about alcohol that are holding you back. Put them around your computer screen so you can see them throughout the day. Continually challenge them.

STEP 2 – ONE YEAR FROM NOW

Pretend it's one year from now. You have just lived the greatest year of your life. Write down what happened in that year and sell yourself on it every day.

STEP 3 – OLD & NEW IDENTITY

Write down the person you want to become by listing:

- The old traits and values to banish from your identity. For example, 'I am a drinker'.

- The traits that you want to keep. For example, 'I am hard working'.

- The new traits and values to build on or add to your identity. For example, 'I am sober.'

- Write down your compelling future.

STEP 4 – QUIT LIT

Submerge yourself in Quit Lit. There are endless streams of Quit Lit out there, including this book! The alcohol-free living books that helped me build my argument against alcohol and re-condition my mind of the falsehood that 'alcohol is good for you' are, Annie Grace's *Naked Mind* and, my favourite, Craig Beck's *Alcohol Lied To Me*.

Possibly one of the best books ever written, which also had a huge influence on me from an 'I can do this' perspective, was Victor Frankl's *Man's Search for Meaning*. I should also mention Anthony Robbins' *Awaken the Giant Within*.

The podcasts that made a difference are: *The Daily Stoic*; *The 5AM Miracle*; Rich Roll; and Tara Brach.

STEP 5 – QUOTES THAT RESONATE

If a quote resonates with you, write it down. Put it somewhere you can see it. Read it every day. There were many quotes that helped me 'change my mind'. Here are two of my favourites:

'Two roads diverged in a wood, and I, I took the one less travelled by, and that has made all the difference.' Robert Frost

'I am the master of my fate, I am the captain of my soul.' William Ernest Henley

KEY LEARNINGS

- Life is a gigantic self-fulfilling prophecy. We spend our whole life telling stories about ourselves. These stories become real and are often full of limiting beliefs.

- Train the voice in your head (your ego) through mindfulness to behave like a scout and look objectively at facts about alcohol.

- Relentlessly read new information from Quit Lit, supporting the new you and the story that alcohol is poison and kills you. It is not fun or a relaxant.

- Create new pathways in your mind by thinking your new story over and over again just like Thoreau tells us in *Pathways of the Mind*. 'One more won't hurt' becomes 'One will hurt you'.

- The new you does not react to events – it responds. This is a key difference.

- To make a shift in your identity you need to redefine yourself. You are not your behaviour. You are your beliefs.

- Create a compelling future for yourself and live it.

CHAPTER 13
CRAVINGS & WILLPOWER

Cravings and willpower are two core pieces of the jigsaw that holds the secret to becoming alcohol-free.

MY STORY

I realised early on that I only needed to use willpower for long enough to build a new habit. Once the new habit takes over, the need for willpower goes away. This is echoed by Gary Keller in his book *The One Thing*, in which he says, 'Success is actually a short race – a sprint fuelled by discipline just long enough for habit to kick in and take over.'

I'd failed hundreds of times to get past Day One because I used the willpower-only method to fight my bad habit. I was not changing my beliefs. I was just fighting the belief that 'I am a drinker'.

With a belief change to 'I am a non-drinker', I ONLY need willpower when a craving is triggered and ONLY in the first few weeks. It's sounds so simple – because it is. Cravings soon start to get less frequent when you have an underlying belief change.

TWO VOICES

I looked at cravings and willpower as two voices inside my head. The craving voice was telling me, 'A drink would be great!' – on a hot summer's day, after work, with a meal or at the airport. This is my primitive brain, my ego, telling me it's OK to do what I want and to go ahead and satisfy a short-term desire.

This craving voice is very much part of the habit loop. It is triggered by many things, such as a location (walking past a pub), time (end of the working day), or my emotional state (stressed, happy, celebratory).

The willpower voice, or self-control, was saying the opposite: 'No, you have a longer-term goal'. It was telling me not to drink. It was my determination. It was my self-discipline. The willpower voice was the voice of the new belief, the new pathway I was building.

So there we have it, two voices, two sides having a discussion, a fight in my head. I was battling against myself. Wow! No-one else is involved. Just me.

The craving versus willpower battle was like self-inflicted anxiety. I tell myself I want something but I also tell myself I can't have it. The only way the new me can win, is to hold my ground, realise what's happening, and accept that it will pass.

The craving voice took me away from the present. It took me to the past where I reminisced on how great drinking is, and the future where I look forward to drinking again. Until my new belief was firmly established, it was willpower I had to rely upon to get me back to the now.

Put very simply, I was taking on my ego. I was testing my ability to resist temptation of my short-term desires for a longer-term goal.

THE ROLE OF WILLPOWER

The pathway I took to alcohol-free living is based on changing my beliefs but willpower still had an important part to play.

I can't stress enough that my approach was NOT willpower centred. I had tried that approach many times before and it never worked for me, or for millions of others.

Approaching it solely with willpower is either doomed to fail or subscribing you to a life of constant battle with yourself, putting yourself through unimaginable mental pain and suffering.

Over the first few weeks, when your new beliefs are starting to take hold, you need willpower to fight off the cravings. Willpower was critical in the early days but less and less so as my new beliefs became solidified and the new pathways in my mind, and ways of thinking, became established.

WHAT I LEARNT

CRAVINGS ARE LIKE WAVES

A metaphor that worked for me and helped me quash my cravings was likening them to waves crashing on a beach. I would go down to the seaside two or three times a week in the first few weeks of stopping drinking to watch the waves. Each craving is like a wave. Each has a start. Some are bigger than others. Some last longer than others. What they all have in common is they all end when they crash on the shore.

I found this a very pleasant and fun way to think about and deal with cravings, knowing they will pass.

UNPACKING WILLPOWER

Author Dan Millman says that willpower is the key to success. Successful people strive, no matter what they feel, by applying their will to overcome apathy, doubt or fear.

Kelly McGonigal in her book *The Willpower Instinct* says that willpower is comprised of three things: 'I won't power', 'I willpower'; and 'I want power'.

According to positive psychologist Catarina Lino, 'Self-control or willpower appears to be a better predictor of academic achievement than intelligence. It is also a stronger determinant of effective leadership than charisma and more important for marital satisfaction than empathy.' She says, 'People with greater willpower are: happier; healthier; more satisfied in their relationships; wealthier and further ahead in their careers; and more able to manage stress, deal with conflict and overcome adversity. Most of us would be closer to achieving all our goals if we focused on improving our willpower.'

WHERE IS WILLPOWER LOCATED IN YOUR BRAIN

I am a firm believer that the more you know about something, the easier it becomes to understand it and influence it. Psychologists have identified the area of the brain that allows us to regulate our behaviour as the Prefrontal Cortex (PFC). This area does not fully develop until around our mid-20s, which explains perfectly why otherwise sensible teenagers take part in high-risk behaviours, even though they understand the consequences.

The importance of the PFC is highlighted when you look at what happens when it is damaged. In the 19th century, a man called Phineas Gage had an accident at work, which resulted in his PFC being cut away when an iron rod penetrated his skull. He survived but had massive changes to his personality. Before the accident, friends and family described him as quiet and respectful. His physician Dr. Harlow described the differences as, 'The balance between his intellectual faculties and his animal propensities seems to have been destroyed. He is fitful, irreverent, impatient of restraint or advice when it conflicts with his desires...' When he lost his PFC, Gage also lost his willpower.

There are other ways we can inhibit our PFC, and therefore our willpower, without cutting it off. These include being drunk. So, after the first drink, it becomes easier to have the second, and the third, and so on, because our willpower is being diminished and we start to focus on our impulses, not our long-term goals. So, if you don't inhibit your PFC, you will have more willpower.

HOW TO STRENGTHEN YOUR WILLPOWER

We rely on willpower to exercise, diet, save money, quit smoking, stop drinking, overcome procrastination and ultimately accomplish any of our goals. It impacts every area of our lives.

Look at willpower as a resource. It can be strengthened like a muscle, stored and used when you need it.

It's a bit like the latest F1 racing cars. The driver is able to get a few more miles per hour out of the car, enabling them to pull off an overtake from the additional battery energy saved as they go around the track.

According to Catarina Lino, you can strengthen your willpower through several channels, including improving your self-awareness, meditating, exercise and a healthy diet.

Baba Shiv, Professor of Marketing at Stanford Business School, found that distracted people are more likely to give in to temptation. For example, distracted shoppers are more sensitive to instore promotions, and more likely to purchase items that were not on their shopping list. From a drinking perspective, you can improve the effectiveness of your willpower if you can identify the triggers that make you want to drink so you can prepare and be ready – it won't be a surprise.

Training your brain for better self-control, through mindfulness practice, is one of the best ways to increase willpower. Meditation has a powerful effect on a wide range of skills that relate to self-control, such as attention, focus, stress management, impulse control and self-awareness. Regular meditators have more grey matter in the prefrontal cortex and other areas of the brain responsible for self-awareness.

I can 100% vouch for exercising as a sure-fire way of improving willpower. I walk at least 9km every day and it definitely has an effect on all parts of my life. I can honestly say that I have more willpower because my longer-term goals have become much more centre stage and more important than my short-term gains or desires. Of course, I think I'd love a biscuit with a cup of tea, or chips for lunch some days, but I ask myself, what would a person with the goals that I have do? What would a person who walks 9km every day, who wants to be fit and healthy, do? In most cases, this is enough to have one biscuit instead of two!

Stress shifts your brain to a reward-seeking state – whatever makes you happy at the moment will become a fixation. This is why people who are stressed are more likely to reach for a cigarette, a drink or fast food. According to the American Psychology Association (APA), the most common stress coping strategies are also the least effective ones: gambling, smoking, playing video games, surfing the internet, or watching TV and movies (for more than 2 hours). Some of the most effective stress-relief strategies are: exercising or playing sports, praying or attending religious service, reading, listening to music, spending time with loved ones, getting a massage, meditating, doing yoga or going out for a walk.

WILLPOWER THROUGHOUT THE DAY

Roy F. Baumeister, the American social psychologist, says that from the moment we wake up until we go to sleep, we are constantly using our willpower. A growing body of research proves that resisting temptations takes a toll on us mentally. Some researchers claim that our willpower, just like a muscle, can get tired if used too much.

Researchers on self-control also advise that muscles can become fatigued when overused in the short term, but over the long-run, they are strengthened by regular exercise.

Similarly, using your self-control frequently and effectively can lead to stronger willpower muscles.

Psychologists also agree that willpower is more plentiful earlier in the day.

STEPS YOU CAN TAKE

STEP 1 – GO TO THE SEASIDE

Sit on the beach and watch the waves crashing. Surf The Urge. If a seaside trip is out of the question, watch a *YouTube* video of waves crashing.

STEP 2 – STRENGTHEN YOUR WILLPOWER

You can do this by:

- Improving your self-awareness, meditating, exercise and eating a healthy diet.
- Understanding the triggers that make you want to drink so you can prepare and be ready.
- Using self-control frequently.

KEY LEARNINGS

- Cravings and willpower are two core pieces of the jigsaw that holds the secret to becoming alcohol-free.
- You ONLY need willpower when a craving is triggered, and ONLY in the first few weeks.
- Cravings soon start to get less frequent when you have an underlying belief change.
- Cravings and willpower are two voices inside your head. Voice One is the craving and it's telling you that 'you want something'. Voice Two is willpower or self-control and it's saying 'no, you have a longer-term goal'.
- A craving is like a wave. Each has a start. Some are larger than others. Some last longer than others. What they all have in common is that they end when they crash on the shore.

CHAPTER 14
WRITE IT DOWN

Writing things down is a great way of learning. If I just watch a video, listen to a podcast or read a book, I am less likely to remember the details than if I write it down. There is something about transferring the idea onto paper through your own hand. It works for me and I am sure it will work for you.

MY STORY

From Day One, I kept a handwritten A5 journal, covering each day of my journey. By the end of the 365 days, I had four volumes or around 800 pages of my thoughts. When my 365 days were up, I continued with my journaling and as I write this, I am on volume six.

My journal captures what I am thinking – my hopes, fears, beliefs, values, purpose, goals and dreams. It is a powerful reminder of how far I have come. When I read the entries, I can see how I am evolving and growing.

Here are a few examples taken from the first few days and months of my AF journey:

Day One

'Reprioritise alcohol in my life. Replace with other habits. Watch the daily video, join the *One Year No Beer* Facebook group, listen to alcohol-free podcasts, read alcohol-free books.'

'Why am I taking this challenge? To be healthier. To lose weight. To not look like I am an alcoholic. To have better and more fulfilling relationships with those close to me.'

'Short-term – feel better, have better skin, be less stressed. Longer-term – sleep better, snore less, look better, be calm and collected.'

All that would have been lost if I had not written it down. I went on to achieve all those objectives, but if I had not journaled them I would probably have forgotten them and almost certainly would not have achieved them.

Day Three

'Need to create a challenge for myself – daily 1km run. Learn a song a day on the guitar.'

'Woke up with the following positives. Poison feeling in mouth getting better. Less pins and needles in my feet and hands. Much more awake. Feel alive.'

God, what was I doing to myself for all those years? Again, looking at this with today's mindset and beliefs, I was in such a mess, letting alcohol control me and affect my life. Reading this entry reinforces my decision never to go back to drinking alcohol.

Day 18 – Christmas Day

'Got up at 0730 and went for 1km jog with Jonesey (my dog). Time 10 minutes, 14 seconds.'

'Choose the right path. Turn left, go back to where I came from. Turn right, continue on my alcohol-free journey.'

Wow, this is pretty powerful stuff. Christmas Day jogging! Reaffirming the path. I was definitely metamorphosising into the new me.

Day 60

'Happiness is not a destination, it's a cultivation.'

'Smile. It makes me happy.'

'I am in charge of my own destiny, how I feel and what I respond to. Therefore, I can change everything. Focus on my goals and the way will appear.'

You can see, in just these few entries, how I am changing. This is one of the core powers of journaling.

Reflecting on all this, the most important thing a journal gives me, above everything else, is accountability.

These pages list my goals and objectives, my mantras. They are there in black and white. Writing it down has a huge power and it was a vital ingredient to my successful journey.

If you are worried that you won't have anything to write about and you'll be struggling to fill the pages, don't. It's not about the quantity, it's about the quality. I very rarely wrote more than two pages for each day. However, over the year, this turned into 800-plus pages, which have provided me with a lot of content for this book.

I'd written several diaries as a child, and many family holiday diaries when the children were growing up. All my diaries are handwritten – pen to paper. Call me old-fashioned but I prefer this to typing on my iMac. Of course, it does not matter what pen you use as long as it's got ink, but I do use a gold Montblanc, a gift from a special person a few years ago. It's like the difference between drinking tea out of a mug and a bone china cup. It just tastes better. Beliefs are everything!

For me, pen to paper feels like the words are coming straight out through the pen onto the paper. There's no spellcheck or auto-correct. If you delete something, you have to put a line through it – but it's still there.

I think it's more creative than using a keyboard. It's as if the thoughts just spill out better through a pen. This may be, however, because I cannot type very quickly!

CALENDAR ON THE FRIDGE

As well as the diaries, I also use a wall calendar as a form of journaling. On Day One, I printed off an A4 calendar with the whole year on one page, so I could cross off the days as I journeyed to Day 365.

This wall calendar was strategically placed on the fridge door – the old gateway to ice-cold booze. This was where all the alcoholic 'goodies' such as cold wine and beer, plus the ice cubes for that large nightcap, hung out.

This messy piece of paper became central to my journey, a daily reminder of my success, of how far I had come. Each cross was a loaded reminder of the cravings that I had conquered, the days I had notched up.

Each day, the first thing I did on entering the kitchen was put a cross in the box for that day, making it a form of self-fulfilling prophecy that I had *already* achieved the day without alcohol.

It all sounds so simple, but do not underestimate the power of one of these wall calendars. I was and am 'AF and loving it' every day.

MANTRAS

The final part of my journaling portfolio was a series of Post-it notes that I put around my house and office, mainly on the bottom of my computer screen, as a daily reminder. I call these my mantras.

If I came across a saying or quote that I liked and that I thought would make my journey easier, I would write it onto a Post-it. I put it where I could see it each day and occasionally said it out loud.

Try it – although it sounds crazy, it really works.

WHAT I LEARNT

I read that mantras originated in religious ceremonies, sung by priests. As well as quotes or sayings, mantras can be just words, which I attached greater meaning to. I find them to be powerful tools to help me meditate. I use them if I feel the need to 'get into the zone' quickly. I simply softly say the word 'relax' on the in breath and 'now' on the out breath. This creates a trance-like state. You should try it.

STEPS YOU CAN TAKE

STEP 1 – JOURNALING

- Purchase a good quality journal. Ideally something that will last and look good on your bookshelf.

- Build some time into each day to write in your journal – make it a habit. I always write my journal straight after breakfast. It just becomes routine.

- Write down what you have learnt and what resonates with you.

- Read your journal. Get into a routine of reading it at the end of each day or the end of each week.

STEP 2 – CALENDARS

- Print off a wall calendar. There are loads online. Stick it on your fridge door and mark off each day as you progress through the first week, month and year of your challenge.

STEP 3 – MANTRAS

- If you see a good quote, or read something that resonates with you, write it down on a sticky note and put it on your computer screen or bathroom mirror – somewhere you can see it and read it regularly.

- Softly say the word 'relax' on the in breath and 'now' on the out breath when you start your meditation. This quickly creates a trance-like state.

KEY LEARNINGS

- A journal captures what you are thinking: your hopes, fears, beliefs, values, purpose, goals and dreams. It is a powerful reminder of how far you have come. When you read the entries, you can see how you are evolving and growing.

- The most important thing a journal gives you, above everything else, is accountability.

- Recognise the good things you already have in your life. The more you think this way, the happier you become.

- Writing things down is a great way of learning.

- A one-page wall calendar was central to my journey, a daily reminder of my success, of how far I had come. Each cross was a loaded reminder of the cravings that I had conquered, the days I had notched up.

- If I came across a saying or quote that I liked and that I thought would make my journey easier, I wrote it onto a Post-it and put it where I could see it each day and occasionally say it out loud.

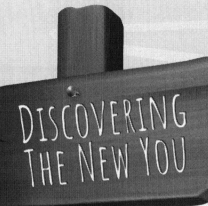

DISCOVERING THE NEW YOU

The First Few Weeks

DISCOVERING THE NEW YOU: THE FIRST FEW WEEKS

The world is soaked in alcohol. Everywhere you look is touched by alcohol – TV, cinema, social media, work, celebrities, friends, family, holidays, eating, sport, birthdays, deaths and marriages. You name it...

Stopping drinking is the gateway to the real you. Stopping this one habit will unleash the best possible you. You will be able to do anything you want to. This one change can lead to a new life, new connections, and a fitter, calmer you.

In this section, I explore the major things I did that propelled me forward on the trajectory to well-being and finding my authentic self.

I cover mindfulness and meditation, gratitude, alcohol-free drinks and how I moved my body clock and get the best out of the early hours of the morning – a freedom alcohol-free gives you.

CHAPTER 15
MEDITATION & MINDFULNESS: LIVING IN THE PRESENT – IT'S A GIFT

It's difficult, if not impossible, to be fully present and give full attention to what is happening now in your life if you are under the influence of any drug, particularly alcohol. An old Zen saying suggests, 'You should sit in meditation for 20 minutes every day – unless you're too busy. Then you should sit for an hour.'

MY STORY

When I stopped drinking, I needed to address all my fears, everything that was holding me back. I needed to become strong and move forward. I simply could not have done it without meditation and mindfulness.

At the beginning of this alcohol-free journey, I harboured limiting beliefs about meditation and mindfulness. I thought it would be a weird thing to do. It was something monks did! Maybe it was just my generation. I realise now that this was just a defence mechanism because I did not understand their power and how effective they could be for my health. If I knew then what I know now, I would probably be a Zen master today!

KUNG FU PANDA HELPED ME DOUBLE MY LIFE

I was, like many people, similar to the character Mr. Duffy, in James Joyce's *Dubliners*, who 'lived a short distance from his body'.

To put it very simply, I was not present. I was, most of the time, somewhere else. Thinking about the past or the future but rarely in the present moment, or the now. Alcohol does this to you. When you drink, you leave the now and go somewhere else. That's pretty much the plan. You drink to relax, have fun, escape – well, you *think* you do.

When I started to understand the implications of this powerful life skill called mindfulness, it very quickly changed my life and was like a nuclear weapon in the arsenal I was using to change my beliefs, my story and my road towards a much happier life.

The road to Damascus – 'I have seen the light' – moment came when I was walking along a country lane on one of my 9KM BY 9AM walks. I was playing around with the words of Master Oogway from the movie *Kung Fu Panda*: 'The past is history, the future is a mystery and today is a gift and that is why we call it the present.' I love that line. But the words became so real when I looked back down the road I had just come from (the past) and forward to where I was potentially going (the future) and where I was (the now). Eureka! I understand it. It is my body that is always in the now. It can't be in the past or the future. So, it is only my mind that wanders and takes me backwards or forwards. And I can control this through mindfulness and meditation.

Not only would I be happier and content if I lived as much as possible in the present, but I could also double the amount of time I had on this planet. But how?

Studies show we spend up to 50% of our time either worrying about the past or anxious about something that has not yet happened! Through meditation and mindfulness practices, I was learning how to control my thoughts and live more in the now – not the past or the future. By doing this, I could effectively save 50% of my time, thereby doubling the amount of time I have!

A recent study by Harvard University researchers tracked the thoughts and activities of several thousand volunteers. It found that almost half the time their thoughts were not related to the activity they were engaged in. In other words, for 50% of our time, we are not present. They also found that we're happiest when we are present and focused on exactly what we're doing, whether that's having a conversation, walking down the street or doing the dishes.

USE IT IN YOUR DAY-TO-DAY LIFE

Meditation works for me so I wholeheartedly recommend giving it a try. You will have a richer experience of the world, improve your well-being, have more and better connections with others, and gain an understanding of those negative patterns that hold you back from achieving your full potential for happiness.

I learnt how to do it, so you can as well. Once you have mastered this, you can use it in your day-to-day life. If you feel yourself worrying about the future or having anxiety over the past – take yourself to the now. The now is where things happen. They don't happen in the past!

Mentally, I would now label myself as a calm person – certainly not a term I would have used before I stopped drinking. Without a doubt, the effects of alcohol made me short-tempered and on edge. It's amazing how, even after one or two days not drinking, these effects start to subside.

The deeper I go into this alcohol-free journey, the more contemplative I become. Anger and quick-reaction responses become less and less. The way I respond to the things that happen to me has become more controlled, calmer, more thoughtful and more empathetic.

The Stoic philosophers said that we don't control the world around us but we do control how we respond. The saying, 'It's not what happens to you, it's the way you react that matters', or versions of it, have been used by many great minds over the years. Being alcohol-free definitely makes you calmer, and practising mindfulness and meditation makes you the calmest you can possibly be.

I experimented with meditation, once or twice a week, in the early months of going alcohol-free. But it was not until around six months in, that I started to meditate as I walked 9KM BY 9AM every day. It became second nature to walk down the country lanes or along the country paths focusing on my breath and clearing my mind, finding the space between my thoughts.

Initially, I listened to guided meditations by Tara Brach, which are available for a voluntary donation from her website or free if you have a limited budget. I still do this once a week, but I mainly guide myself these days. Once you get into the swing of it, it's pretty much like second nature.

WHAT I LEARNT

There were several books that helped me fully understand this new power I was developing, including: *The Power of Now* by Eckhart Tolle, *Aware* by Dan Siegel and *10% Happier* by Dan Harris. I also listened to podcasts from Tara Brach and Jack Kornfield, as well as the *One Year No Beer* course *Mindfulness 10 – Live Life Better*.

DEFINING MINDFULNESS VS MEDITATION

Lots of books and articles talk about mindfulness and meditation but definitions are not readily available.

In fact, it is all pretty straightforward, and you don't have to meditate to be mindful.

Mindfulness is a non-judgmental awareness of your thoughts, sensations, surroundings and emotions. Meditation is just one tool for developing mindfulness, but it isn't the only tool.

TYPES OF MEDITATION

There's no right or wrong way to meditate and there are several popular types of meditation practice to choose from. For me, movement meditation is my favourite as it fits perfectly with my 9KM BY 9AM morning walks.

Movement meditation is most famous for yoga but also includes walking, gardening, tai chi, and other forms of movement. This is an active form of meditation where the movement guides you into a deeper connection with your body and the present moment. Movement meditation is good for people who find peace in action and want to develop body awareness.

There are many other main types. These include guided meditation, mindfulness meditation or present moment meditation, spiritual meditation, focused meditation, mantra meditation, transcendental meditation, progressive relaxation or body scan meditation, loving-kindness meditation or metta meditation and visualisation meditation or vipassana meditation.

BRINGING FEAR INTO THE PRESENT MOMENT

When we bring mindfulness and compassion to our fears, we can reconnect. When we experience fear, it's normally because we are worrying about the future. We are not present.

Fear could be the worry that 'I might cave in to a craving and start drinking again'. It can be lots of things. Fear takes us away from the real world. It takes us away from being in the present because we're worrying about the future. To get back to the present, you need to use mindfulness and compassion to address the fear. Yoda said, 'Named must your fear be, before banish it you can.'

By addressing fear, by processing it, by not running away from it, you bring it into the present.

THE WINDOW OF REACTION

Learning how to free your mind through meditation is such an amazing tool – and so simple. By learning how to be more present, you are less likely to get caught up in stories in your head or fall into reactive patterns of behaviour like arguing and making poor choices.

The biggest thing I learnt from mindfulness is how to build the 'window of reaction', that is, the time between stimulus and your reaction to a stimulus. The stimulus could be, 'It's a sunny evening and I fancy a glass of wine'. One reaction might be to go ahead and have one. Another, and the best course, would be to do something else, like learn a new song on the guitar. If you can control the reaction to a stimulus, you are pretty much in control of your destiny.

STEPS YOU CAN TAKE

STEP 1 – DECIDE YOU'RE GOING TO GIVE IT A GO

Meditation is like a workout for your mind. I think of it as building my mind muscle. Just exercising my mind for five to ten minutes per day has a massive effect. The ability to train myself to clear my mind of past or future thoughts, and just think of what is now, helps me think before I react.

It's best to start in small increments of time, even five or ten minutes, and grow from there. Pedram Shojai, author of *The Urban Monk* says, 'Sit consistently for 20 minutes a day and do this for 100 days straight. Couple that with an additional two to five minutes of meditation throughout the day to break up the chaos, and you will soon be feeling the benefits.'

STEP 2 – PRACTISE! PRACTISE! PRACTISE!

Practising mindfulness throughout your everyday life can help to train the mind to focus on the present.

Once you've installed meditation, you can go to it any time and build your mind muscle. So, if you get stuck in a queue at a bank or in a traffic jam, or you simply have a spare five minutes – meditate!

Here are just a few examples of how you can be mindful in every situation you find yourself in. By doing this, you start to control how you react to the things that happen to you. I've tried all of these and they work.

* *Drinking tea or coffee*: Smell and examine your tea or coffee before taking a slow sip. Close your eyes and wholly feel and taste the liquid on your tongue before swallowing. Feel the warmth of the cup in your hands.

* *Taking a shower*: Think about what the water feels like as it hits your skin.

* *Scanning your body*: Take a moment to close your eyes and tune into your body. Start at your toes and move up, observing each body part until you reach the top of your head. Be curious about what you find, noticing any tension, lightness, heat, pain or other sensations. Notice if the mind wanders and creates stories about those feelings. If so, see if you can bring the mind back to the sensations without judging them.

* *Sunrise or sunset*: Take in the unique colours and try to notice something you've never spotted before. Is there a cloud shape that reminds you of something or someone? What colours do you see? How does the air temperature change once the sun dips below the horizon?

STEP 3 – BRING 'RAIN' TO YOUR MEDITATION

When you're meditating ask yourself the simple question 'What is happening right now in my life?'

This is a great way to bring to the front of your mind the issues you think you might have. This could be drinking. It could be addictions or it could be relationships.

Try Tara Brach's RAIN approach to meditation. This is an acronym for:

Recognise the issue you have.

Allow whatever it is to be. Don't brush it under the carpet.

Investigate what's causing it. Have an open discussion with yourself about it.

Nurture the issue and explore ways of dealing with it.

By using the RAIN method, I changed my beliefs not only about alcohol but about all my anxieties.

KEY LEARNINGS

- Mindfulness is a non-judgmental awareness of your thoughts, sensations, surroundings and emotions.

- Meditation is just one tool for developing mindfulness but it isn't the only tool.

- The human brain is more powerful than the most powerful supercomputer created to date. But get this – it does not come with an instruction manual. We have to work out how it operates by ourselves. Meditation and mindfulness are like keys that help us unlock our brains so we can access the instruction manual and start to learn to live our best life in the short time we have.

- It's difficult, if not impossible, to be fully present and give full attention to what is happening now in your life if you are under the influence of any drug, particularly alcohol.

- When you drink, you leave the now and go somewhere else. That's pretty much the plan. You drink to relax, have fun, escape – well you *think* you do.

- When I started to understand the implications of this powerful life skill called meditation, it very quickly changed my life and was like a nuclear weapon in the arsenal I was using to change my beliefs, my story and my road towards a much happier life.

- There's plenty of evidence supporting the numerous general health and mental, emotional benefits of mindfulness including: lower blood pressure, reduced stress, better sleep, improved emotional regulation, increased focus, enhanced mood, reduced aggression, greater adaptability, healthier ageing process, a greater sense of empathy and connection with others.

- The biggest thing I learnt from mindfulness is how to build the 'window of reaction', that is, the time between stimulus and your reaction to a stimulus.

- Fear takes us away from the real world. It takes us away from being in the present because we're worrying about the future. To get back to the present you need to use mindfulness and compassion to address the fear. Yoda said, 'Named must your fear be, before banish it you can.'

- If you feel yourself worrying about the future or having anxiety over the past, take yourself to the now. The now is where things happen. They don't happen in the past!

- Being alcohol-free definitely makes you calmer. Practising mindfulness and meditation makes you the calmest you can possibly be.

CHAPTER 16
INSTALLING GRATITUDE

The more I found out about gratitude and its powers, the more I built it into my daily life. I initially thought of it like software. I needed to install both a gratitude app and ingratitude protection software that prevented feelings of ingratitude growing inside me. It was like being vaccinated against ingratitude just by being more grateful.

MY STORY

I am now more content than I have been since my teenage years. A major part of the secret to achieving this and staying on the alcohol-free pathway is down to that one word, GRATITUDE. For me, it's a fast lane to well-being, by appreciating what 'you have' as opposed to the things 'you don't have' and understanding what 'enough' means.

Our million-plus-year-old human brain is designed for survival – fight or flight. This is why it's always busy looking for what's wrong. Cultivating gratitude has been proved to prime our brain to look for the good in things – not the bad.

We are all guilty, some more than others, of looking for the bad in things. It is human nature. But life is so much better when you look for the good in things.

The following are a few of the things I did to help me cultivate gratitude and build and strengthen my gratitude muscle.

FOCUS ON THE POSITIVE

One of the things I did to cultivate gratitude and help change my life was simply to write down in a diary or notebook three things that I was grateful for every day. After a month I had over 90, after six months, 500!

By doing this I focused my mind on the positive things in my life. Dr. Martin E. P. Seligman, a psychologist at the University of Pennsylvania, asked people to write down three things that they are grateful for. After 15 days, 92% of people said their happiness had increased.

The more you think this way, the happier you become. Here are just some of mine over a month:

- Sunrise light coming through bedroom window
- Phone calls from my children
- Seeing my dog asleep in my office
- My wife making me a smoothie
- New guitar day
- Pizza ovens
- Walking in the woods with my dog
- Saturday mornings
- Sunday mornings
- All mornings
- Cold showers
- Long walks
- Roast potatoes
- Sound of rain on window
- My garden
- New grass
- Led Zeppelin
- New rake
- Having dinner cooked for me

- Alpacas
- Walking around the streets where I grew up
- My mum
- Hot cup of tea after a morning walk
- Seeing an old man walking along the road each morning going to collect his daily newspaper
- Buying a newspaper at the weekend
- Learning to box
- Red pillar boxes
- Imperial mints
- Rich Roll podcast
- Breathing hot air out of my mouth on a cold morning so it creates a steam effect
- Fields covered in frost
- Horses running freely
- Finding someone's phone and returning it
- Florentines
- The Post Office
- Marmalade on toast
- Reflections in puddles
- Thick socks in winter
- Working out outside
- The acknowledgement from other drivers who I let pull out in front of me onto a busy road
- Birds singing
- Cleaning rust off steel with a wire brush

GRATITUDE LETTERS

Seligman also tested the impact of writing and personally delivering a letter of gratitude to someone special who had never been properly thanked for his or her kindness.

He found that participants immediately exhibited a huge increase in happiness scores with benefits lasting for a month.

You should try this – I did. I handwrote a 500-word letter to my mother, thanking her for being such a kind mother. I found a quiet moment when we were alone and sitting down. I can tell you now this was a pivotal moment and one of the most emotional experiences of my life. It made me cry with happiness to tell her how important she was to me and how grateful I am that she is my mother. This is the stuff people normally spill out in a eulogy after their loved one has gone and it's too late to tell them all the things they really wanted to say. The effect of this experience lasted ages and has strengthened the bond between us.

If you take anything from this chapter of the book, take this advice and write a letter and read it to your loved one today. It will change your life – and theirs.

ACTS OF KINDNESS

I perform at least one act of kindness a day. An example of this is doing a good deed for someone.

I feel just as good, if not better, when I give someone a gift as opposed to receiving a gift. This act could be as simple as holding a door open for someone.

What's going on here is that you are tapping into gratitude and priming your brain.

MEDITATION - INSTALLING GRATITUDE

I found meditating to be one of the most basic ways to gladden my mind just by reflecting on where the goodness is in my life. Let's say it's 'I love walking and being in nature'. You have to really let yourself feel the gratitude and then stay with that feeling. Our memory takes in information that's difficult and negative and remembers it for a really long time, but the positive feelings aren't as 'sticky'. So, in order to remember gratitude and have it become a part of you, when you feel grateful, stay with the feeling for 15 to

30 seconds. Neuroscience shows this works. Rick Hanson calls it 'installing the trait of gratitude'.

SAY IT OUT LOUD

When I feel grateful, I say what I appreciate out loud. You can write it or say it, because the expressing brings it through your body and creates a fuller experience

WHAT I LEARNT

POSITIVE PSYCHOLOGY

Positive psychology research shows that gratitude is strongly and consistently associated with greater happiness. Gratitude helps people feel positive emotions, relish good experiences, improve their health, deal with adversity, and build strong relationships.

IMAGINE IF YOU LOST EVERYTHING

The power and benefits of gratitude are not a new thing. Gratitude is a major pillar of Buddhism, as well as being one of the main principles of Stoicism, a philosophy from 2,000+ years ago.

The Stoics said you should appreciate and be grateful for what you have. A quick way to see the power of this, is to try and understand what your life would be like if you did not have the things in your life like family, friends, a pet, hot showers, a roof over your head, and so on. You should not take this wealth for granted.

Marcus Aurelius, a Roman Emperor and famous Stoic thinker, said, 'When you arise in the morning think of what a privilege it is to be alive, to think, to enjoy, to love'. Epicurus, another famous Stoic, said, 'Do not spoil what you have by desiring what you have not; remember that what you now have was once among the things you only hoped for.'

THE GRATEFUL VIEW

According to Orion Philosophy, gratitude is a way in which we see the world around us. There are perceived to be two extreme views of the world. The Grateful View: I'm not owed anything; we have been given the opportunity to experience life, to create, to think, to build relationships. There are many people who have less than I have, and most of what I have would be missed if it were taken away from me. The Ungrateful View: I deserve more. I have a lot of things, but I really want to have a bigger house, better car, and more money. I get jealous when I see people with things that I want, and it makes me want them even more.

One of these views helps build a mindset of enjoying what you have, being grateful for the life you lead, and building a resilience against feelings of envy, entitlement and dissatisfaction. The other creates a mindset that's prone to jealousy, entitlement, dissatisfaction and a life that's always looking forward to the future, rather than enjoying what you have in the present.

WHAT IS ENOUGH?

It all boils down to knowing when you have enough. When you have enough, you are no longer on the hamster wheel. Knowing the meaning of enough gives you a feeling of calmness, powered by the fact that you have been released from desire and the need to compare yourself to others.

There's a story in the book, *Stillness Is The Key* by Ryan Holiday, that exemplifies this. It's about the writers Kurt Vonnegut and Joseph Heller who went to a party at the magnificent home of a billionaire. Vonnegut questioned Heller about how it felt to realise that the person who hosted the party had possibly earned more that exact day than Heller's book, Catch-22, had made in its entire history. Heller answered by saying that he had something the billionaire would never have, which is the understanding that he had enough. What Heller meant was that he was content with what he had accomplished. If you see yourself desiring for more, remember Heller's contented acceptance of enough.

WHAT STOPS US FROM FEELING GRATEFUL?

What stops us from appreciating friends, family or the natural world around us?

Tara Brach says that for many of us, it's that we're on our way to somewhere else – we're not in the present moment, we're moving through, in some way, trying to get the next cup of coffee or trying to get the next bit of approval from somebody. We're not really here to take in what's right here.

SIX PILLARS

Another influential interview I heard on gratitude is by yoga guru Raghunath Cappo who talks about the six powerful principles to rewire your life and find happiness through acting in a loving way. His six commandments are:

I will not criticise – discern; don't condemn

I am tolerant

I take no offence – forgive immediately and completely

I am quick to apologise

I see the good in others and I let them know it

I am grateful and I keep a tally of my blessings

DEFINING HAPPINESS

I don't think I'd ever really defined happiness to myself. Moments when I laugh and feel joy are beautiful but are just one element of happiness.

Positive psychology states that well-being encapsulates the various dimensions of 'happiness' and includes engagement, relationships, meaning and accomplishment. It's not just about positive emotions of laughter or buying something new.

I was chasing the wrong things in search of happiness. Material things such as guitars, cars, holidays and new clothes gave me momentary bursts of happiness, but I found that meaning and relationships help me to be happy for a lifetime.

So when I think of gratitude, I think about all the things in my life that make up well-being.

By getting caught up in the emotions of stress, fear, anger, frustration, overwhelm, sadness or worry, I am missing my true spirit. The two that probably messed up my life the most were fear and anger. Gratitude helps me get over this.

STEPS YOU CAN TAKE

Science has proven that we can train ourselves to go into emotional states of appreciation and gratitude and when we do, we change our body's biochemistry by tapping into gratitude. We prime our brain to find the good in things.

STEP 1 – BUILD YOUR GRATITUDE MUSCLE

To cultivate gratitude and build and strengthen your gratitude muscle, do the following:

Focus on the positive – Write down in a diary or notebook three things that you are grateful for every day. Do this for a month.

Gratitude letters – Write and personally deliver a letter of gratitude to someone special. Tell them how much they mean to you and how grateful you are for them being in your life. Sit down with them and read it out loud.

Acts of kindness – Perform at least one act of kindness a day.

Pause and be grateful – When you see something you are grateful for, get into the habit of pausing and savouring.

Gratitude meditation – When you feel grateful, stay with the feeling for 15 to 30 seconds.

Say it out loud – When you feel grateful, say what you appreciate out loud.

STEP 2 – IMAGINE IF YOU LOST EVERYTHING

The Stoics said you should appreciate and be grateful for what you have. A quick way to see the power of this is to try and understand what your life would be like if you did not have the things in your life like family, friends, a pet, hot showers, a roof over your head, and so on.

Make a list of the things that you have that you are grateful for.

STEP 3 – WHAT IS YOUR WORLD VIEW?

Which extreme view of the world do you associate with: the 'grateful view' or the 'ungrateful view'?

STEP 4 – PRIME YOURSELF

Anthony Robbins says that you can't be angry and grateful at the same time. Nor can you be fearful and grateful at the same time. He developed a daily 10-minute practice called PRIMING. I have done this many times and it works:

- Step into a moment you feel grateful for as if you are there.

- See what you saw then now, hear what you heard then now. Fill up with gratitude. Give yourself that gift. For example, it can be a little moment or a great one – the birth of a child, the day you got married, laughing with dad, and so on. Think of three of these moments.

- Feel an inner smile; feel that gratitude cleansing and healing your mind and body.

- Bring it to your heart, then send it to the ones you love: family friends, partners, co-workers, strangers.

KEY LEARNINGS

- By practising gratitude, you will start to feel better about yourself, others will warm to you and you will altogether have a better life!

- Gratitude helps people feel more positive emotions, relish good experiences, improve their health, deal with adversity, and build strong relationships.

- Appreciating and focusing on the things that 'you have' as opposed to the things 'you don't have' is a fast lane to well-being.

- Our million-plus-year-old human brain is designed for survival – fight or flight. This is why it's always busy looking for what's wrong. Cultivating gratitude has been proven to prime our brain to look for the good in things – not the bad.

CHAPTER 17
ALCOHOL-FREE (AF) DRINKS

When I drank alcohol, AF drinks were not something I looked forward to. I did not 'get' what they were about. Why would I want a drink that looks like alcohol but does not have any alcohol in it? To my deluded drinking mind, that was a big waste of money. The fact that I genuinely thought that alcohol was NOT a waste of money, but AF drinks were, is now so laughable!

MY STORY

My recommendation to anyone setting out on the AF journey is to stock up on a few AF drinks, particularly for the first few weeks. I swear by them.

AF drinks make leaving the world of the Alcohol Drinkers' Tribe so much easier. In the early days, I thought of AF drinks in terms of the board game *Snakes & Ladders*. Having an AF drink is landing on the bottom of a ladder; it propels you along the path to AF freedom. Having an alcoholic drink would be landing on a snake's head and sliding back down the AF journey path.

By AF drinks, I mean drinks that are marketed as alcohol look-a-like drinks with zero or tiny amounts of alcohol content. I am not talking about tea or coffee, or soda water, cola or lemonade. By AF drinks, I mean brands like Heineken 0.0, Guinness 0.0, Leffe Blonde 0.0%, Nosecco, Gordon's 0.0.

Looking at my journal, it was on Day Five of my AF journey that I started to understand the importance of these AF drinks. They made everything so much easier in the first few weeks when the journey had only just begun and I was highly prone to cravings. For the last 35 years, I drank alcohol every day so, of course, I was going to think about it. It was great that there was an alternative available.

I had not planned to start the *One Year No Beer Challenge.* I woke up one morning and, still lying in bed, signed up to the challenge via an email marketing message I received via my phone. I had no AF drinks in the house and since the Quit Lit and members of the OYNB *Challenge* social websites were singing their praises, I put them on the list for the next supermarket shop. I stocked up with a few packs of AF lager and a couple of bottles of AF red wine.

On Saturdays, I usually had a glass of wine or a beer watching the football scores in the early evening. On my first alcohol-free Saturday, along came the craving and I crushed it with an AF alternative. This made it easier to keep on the path to my new life. I drank two Peroni Liberas and two Heineken 0.0s – the equivalent of around two pints of AF lager! They were ice-cold and tasted fantastic. The weird thing was that it actually felt like I was drinking alcohol, but I knew that these AF drinks weren't laced with anxiety. Plus, there was no morning-after headache and, to put icing on the cake, they were half the calories.

I had drunk a few AF beers in the past, when I still drank alcohol, but this was different. I decided at that point that one of my defences, when I needed it, was an AF drink which I now knew would make cravings disappear.

DRINKING AF DRINKS WITH AN AF MINDSET

There's a huge difference in the way I perceive AF drinks now I am a non-drinker. They simply serve a different purpose – well, they certainly do for me.

I had bought AF drinks in the past, with the intention of drinking them if I was going to try and stop drinking for a few days. But what normally happened was that I would not stop drinking and these AF beers would hang around in the cupboard or the bottom of the fridge for months. They would either get thrown out because they were out of date, be given to a non-drinking guest, or I would on a rare occasion, drink them. I remember having one at lunchtime when I fancied a beer but could not drink because I was working, but I just did not like them that much. They tasted a little like their alcohol equivalents but never quite hit the spot. As a drinker, my expectation of an alcoholic drink was to get a 'high' feeling from it, which only comes when the alcohol is added!

I was conscious that I did not want to substitute AF drinks, sometimes known as AF alternatives, for alcohol. And I didn't. I suppose this was because somewhere in the back of my mind there was a fear that I might end up drinking AF drinks instead of alcoholic drinks. There is absolutely no rational reason for this. It was an unfounded belief that had crept in. Over time, I realised this, as I broke free of the control alcohol had had over me.

As I progressed past 90 days, and then 365 days, my relationship with AF drinks evolved.

They were initially a crutch, something I needed to lean on to help me crush powerful early cravings. Every time I felt like an alcoholic drink, I had an AF drink. They have never been substitutes because I have never felt in any way addicted to them.

As time went by and the cravings got fewer, and the distance between my old drinking life and my new alcohol-free life became longer, I had less of a need for an AF drink and would find myself naturally making a cup of tea instead. The new pathway of alcohol-free living I had created in my mind was becoming more and more established and my default drink was becoming a 'nice cup of tea'.

Looking at my journal, I was pretty much drinking one or two 33cl bottles of AF beer, or a glass or two of AF red wine, each day in the first month or so.

From a physical perspective, these were just soft drinks, but from a mental perspective they were a powerful alternative to alcoholic beverages.

I still drink them occasionally, normally on weekends or if I am watching sport. But they are the same as a cup of tea to me. I don't crave them. It just gives me a bit more choice and feels like a more adult drink than a glass of squash or milk!

WHAT'S MY TIPPLE?

I soon started sampling most of what was available at the supermarket to find the ones that I liked the best. In my opinion, the quality of these products has come a long way in a few years, driven by the increase in the number of people stopping drinking across the globe.

Almost all the main players in the alcohol world have an AF offering. There is also a very wide range of red, white and rosé wines. There are some decent sparkling wine alternatives, like Nosecco, plus a growing market for zero spirits, including brands like Gordon's, Tanqueray, Martini, Cedars and Seedlip.

My favourite AF drinks are:

Guinness 0.0

When I first tasted this, I was around nine months into the journey. It comes in cans with a widget so when poured, it looks, smells and tastes like a real pint of Guinness you'd be served in a pub. When I had the first sip, I seriously thought I was drinking an alcoholic drink. I had to read the label countless times to makes sure it was AF. I even started to feel a slight high from the dopamine my body was releasing. In the old drinking days, this would be referred to as 'lightweight!', like getting drunk on a cider ice lolly!

Leffe Blonde 0.0 (25cl bottle)

I like this best on a hot summer day, served in a bowl-style glass, mixed with Aldi's Pilsner 0% Lager (33cl bottle).

Nosecco

I'll drink this on a special occasion or if we're having a 'posh' meal or Sunday roast. It just feels better with food than a Diet Coke.

Fever-Tree (20cl cans)

Any flavour as they're all excellent over ice.

Mocktails

I like making the odd mocktail for special occasions or if I just feel like one. I normally pour a couple of Fever-Tree Clementine 20cl cans over ice and add in some Martini Vibrante and a slice of lime and lemon – lovely. In fact, my mouth is watering just writing this down. It's amazing how you can train your mind to like something!

Tea

Probably my go-to drink – around six cups a day, with soya milk.

MAKE USE OF YOUR GLASSWARE!

Being a former drinker meant I had lots of nice glasses and decanters, which would potentially go to waste. So, if I feel like an AF drink, it's normally from a fancy glass.

WHAT I LEARNT

LESS CALORIES

The AF drinks I drink are classified as 'Alcohol-free'.

There are four types of categorisation often used on labels:

- Alcohol-free: no more than 0.05% ABV. This is because some alcohol forms as part of the brewing process. In fact, there is more alcohol content in a banana than an alcohol-free drink.
- De-alcoholised: no more than 0.5% ABV
- Low-alcohol: no more than 1.2% ABV

- Alcoholic: contains more than 1.2% ABV

Alcohol-free drinks tend to contain fewer calories than alcohol-based drinks. So, choosing an alcohol-free drink over alcohol, alongside a balanced diet and exercise, can be useful if you're trying to lose weight.

COST

Alcohol-free drinks are much cheaper than alcohol-based drinks. The AF drinks I drink are under £10 a week. Compared to alcohol, where I was spending around £15 per day, every day. This added up to around £100 a week – or well over £5,000 per annum! Based on 35 years of drinking, I estimate that I spent almost £175,000 on booze!!! It was probably more than that if you add in the things I did under it's influence, so we could be looking at well over a quarter of a million pounds.

ONE IS ENOUGH

One major bonus is that, unlike alcoholic drinks, AF drinks don't make you thirsty. You'd never do a session of AF beers. I have never felt the need to drink more than one or two. Unlike alcohol, one drink does not lead to another as they are neither dehydrating, nor are they making you chase a dopamine hit.

STEPS YOU CAN TAKE

STEP 1 – GIVE THEM A GO

Wherever you are on your alcohol-free journey – contemplating taking a break, reducing alcohol consumption, taking a break, or have stopped drinking alcohol permanently – why not give AF drinks a try?

Most pubs and restaurants now have an AF drink or two on the menu. There is even a growing trend for AF-only bars, which are starting to pop up in large town centres.

STEP 2 – YOUR ALCOHOL CALORIE INTAKE

Towards the end of my drinking days, I was drinking roughly half a bottle of spirits (ABV 40%), seven bottles of wine (ABV 12.5%) and six pints of beer (ABV 5%) each week. Beer has around 200 calories per pint, wine 650 calories per bottle and spirits 1,700 calories per bottle. That's around 6,500 calories a week. That's more than two and half days' worth of my recommended food allowance. No wonder I was overweight.

With AF drinks, I have around 6 x 33cl bottles a week. Each has 76 calories – so around 460 calories a week!

You can work out your own using the Drinkaware calculator at https://www.drinkaware.co.uk/tools/unit-and-calorie-calculator

KEY LEARNINGS

- My recommendation to anyone setting out on the AF journey is to stock up on AF drinks, particularly for the first few weeks.

- AF drinks are marketed as alcohol look-a-like drinks, with zero or tiny amounts of alcohol content.

- AF drinks were initially a crutch to help me crush early cravings.

- For me, AF drinks are not substitutes because I never felt in any way addicted to them.

- The AF drinks I drink are classified as 'Alcohol-free', having 0.05% Alcohol by Volume (ABV) or less.

- There is more alcohol content in a banana than an alcohol-free drink.

- Alcohol-free drinks tend to contain fewer calories than alcohol-based drinks. So, choosing an alcohol-free drink over alcohol, alongside a balanced diet and exercise, could be useful if you're trying to lose weight.

- Unlike alcohol, one AF drink does not lead to another as they are not dehydrating and are not making you chase a dopamine hit.

CHAPTER 18
MOVING YOUR BODY CLOCK

I went from getting five hours of interrupted sleep, packed with anxiety attacks and trips to the loo because I'd drunk too much alcohol and water to combat its effects, to seven hours of non-stop sleeping like a baby. How did I do it? I stopped drinking alcohol.

MY STORY

When I stopped drinking alcohol, I immediately had more energy and woke up earlier, full of life. This happens to the majority of people who stop drinking. I think that in the early days this 'Wide Awake Club' feeling is caused by a comparison your mind and body makes with the old and new you.

When I drank, I would always wake up with a fuzzy feeling. Even if I just had one drink the night before. If I had more than one drink, I would have a hangover, the severity depending on how much I had poured down my throat.

So, if you take away the drink, you're going to immediately feel better in the mornings – but you perceive this 'better feeling' to be probably ten times better than it is because it is relevant to how rubbish you felt after drinking. Perception is everything. This early morning feeling is one of the best feelings I have ever had – the feeling of being ready for the day, excited to get out of bed.

It's like being a kid again. All the energy you had as a child comes flooding back to you once you take alcohol out of your life.

Since I stopped drinking, this feeling has never gone away. Now well into Year Two of no alcohol, the early morning is my favourite time of the day. It's a time when I can get things done. My mother used to say, 'An hour in the morning is worth two later in the day'. How right she was.

THE BEST TRADE I EVER MADE

Analysing why I have been so successful in achieving a level of well-being I never thought I would feel again, I realised that it all came down to a trade I was making on a daily basis.

I was trading time. Without realising it, I was trading the two hours between 9.30pm and 11.30pm for the three hours between 5am and 8am the next day. Basically, I was going to bed earlier and waking up earlier the next day. I was also getting around seven hours of uninterrupted sleep each night.

The reason I was able to get three hours from trading two hours was because alcohol was no longer present in my body. Without the alcohol you feel physically and mentally superior. So, what I could do in three hours as a drinker, I could do in two or less as an alcohol-free superhero!

THE EARLY HOURS

One of the key ingredients that has led to the massive improvement in my well-being is the early hours.

5.30am to 7.30am When I drank, I rarely saw these hours as I used to wake up at around 7am and lie in bed with some form of headache until around 8am. Of course, if I had to be up in London for a meeting, I would get up earlier, but most of the time I rose at 8am.

My office is next door to my home so even though I got up at 8am, I was still in work and at my desk by 8.30am –

most days. But now I was alcohol-free, I was full of life at 5.30am. I had my mojo back. So I was now up and about and I had so much energy I started filling this time with exercise, meditation and planning. In the first month, I set myself a challenge of trying to run or jog one kilometre each morning. This progressed to early morning dog walks and eventually ended up as walking at least 9km followed by home gym workout sessions, and all before 9am.

The trade of swapping alcohol for feeling great, had a further upside of a new time of the day to fill with things that were good for me, like physical activity, meditation and education, through podcasts and books.

I was no longer lying in bed full of self-pity thinking 'poor old me' with my raging hangover.

THE NEW LATE

To be in the 'Wide Awake Club' on an on-going basis I had to trade the time from another part of the day: 9.30pm to 11.30pm. The last few hours of the day were normally spent finishing off a bottle of wine while watching TV. This was dead time. Wasted time. Need I say more. This is a fantastic deal. So I went ahead and did it and have never looked back.

Speaking on the Rich Roll podcast, Joe de Sena, the founder of the obstacle race series Spartan, said that he sets his alarm clock to go to bed not to get out of bed. I love that phrase because it resonates exactly with what I am doing.

Looking at this now through my alcohol-free, loving-life goggles, I was living an extremely unhealthy existence. I had no idea what I was missing. All those sunrises. All those books and podcasts I listened to on all those walks where I got closer to nature and finding myself.

MY NEW TYPICAL DAY

I always thought I was a natural morning person but alcohol took this away from me, along with hundreds of other things. When I finally stopped drinking, I got my love of mornings back. Here is my typical day then and now:

TIME	NEW TYPICAL DAY	OLD TYPICAL DAY
3am	Asleep	Go to the loo in middle of night
4am	Asleep	After checking emails and social media for the past hour fall back to sleep
5am	Wake up naturally, no alarm clock	Asleep
5.20am	Get up, drink water, go to loo, get dressed, feed my cat	Asleep
5.45am	Leave house for 9km walk with my dog	Asleep
7am	Walking	Wake up naturally through feeling anxious and/or stressed about something or alarm goes off
8am	Back from walk, 30-minute workout on punch bag (Tai Chi, Kung Fu), free weights and sit-ups	Get up, shower, get dressed
8.15am		Breakfast – toast
8.30am	Shower, dress	Work/hobbies
8.50am	Breakfast – cereal, fruit	
9am	Work/hobbies	
midday	Lunch	Lunch
12.30pm	Work/hobbies	Work/hobbies
5.30pm		First drinks of evening
6.30pm	Dinner	Dinner

7pm	Read, write book, play piano, play guitar, work out	TV plus snacks throughout the night linked to drinking e.g. salted nuts, crisps
9.30pm	Bed/sleep	
11.30pm	Asleep	Bed/sleep

The shaded areas represent the times I traded.

Major positive changes are:

- Sleeping through the night

- Using the early morning to exercise, learn and train my mind

- Eating within a 9 to 10-hour period, roughly 9am to 7pm

- Feeling wide awake

- Feeling very tired at 9.30pm and falling asleep almost immediately because I have burnt around 1,500 calories during the day through exercise

In the last days of my alcohol drinking life, nothing good was happening in the evening other than drinking and eating snacks, mixed with watching copious amounts of TV.

For me, this trade unlocked my life and allowed me to get fit and learn new things, as opposed to drinking and watching loads of TV – most of which I could not remember anyway!

When I tell this story to others, I have a mixed reaction. A lot of people don't like the mornings; they like a lie-in. There is nothing wrong with that. So did I when I was a drinker.

What I very soon realised, once I went alcohol-free, is that the mornings are the best time of the day.

Being alcohol-free, I now naturally wake up at 5am, wide-eyed and ready for the day ahead because I joined the 'Wide Awake Club'.

ONE SIZE DOES NOT FIT ALL

I fully understand that the time trade I made may sound too rigid, or even unrealistic, to some. Lifestyle and existing commitments might make this change difficult to achieve.

It would be easy to say, 'I can't do this because I like doing things between 9pm and 11.30pm', or 'I just don't want to stop going to the theatre, the cinema, or out with friends to restaurants, in the late evening'. Or your reason could be work related, such as, 'Socialising in the evening is part of my job', or 'I work shifts', or 'I am on call'. It could also be, 'I have a baby or a young child who wakes in the early hours', or 'I have elderly parents who need my assistance at night'.

There will be thousands of reasons why you can't make this trade. I had a stack of reasons that I had used for over 35 years. But I decided that the time had come to look at how I *could do it* and not at why I *couldn't do it*.

This was the trade I made and I understand for others this may not be possible to do in exactly the way I did it. But you just need to make the changes that will work for you in your life. It's your choice, no one else's.

Remember we're talking about real life-changing stuff here. Going alcohol-free is a new world. It's easy to make up reasons to stay. My story shows how I escaped. How I found a way out. How I created an opportunity to jump off the wheel.

If you really want to change your life, if you want it badly enough, then you'll find a way.

WHAT I LEARNT

A CLOSER LOOK AT SLEEP

As soon as I stopped drinking, my sleep improved. I started to fall asleep as soon as my head hit the pillow.

This is because I am more active and because I am not hungover. I am back to how things should be naturally. The normal I'd got used to was based on drinking a litre of neat alcohol each week. Of course I was going to feel better and sleep better if I stopped drinking fuel. What's so hard to understand about that?

However, over the first weeks, there were a few days when I found it hard to sleep, with aches in my legs. It was not painful, just annoying. I'm not sure if this was some form of physical withdrawal, but it soon disappeared when I started exercising regularly.

Other reasons why some people who stop drinking find themselves lying awake at night, include: the liver working overtime getting rid of toxins; missing the sedative affect alcohol can have; a massive drop in the amount of sugar in the body, a stimulant that affects your sleep.

WORKING OUT YOUR OPTIMUM LEVEL OF SLEEP

I worked out the optimum number of sleep hours I needed to be six and a half to seven hours. For the past nine months or so, I've been fast asleep between 10.15pm and 4.45am.

Once you know your optimum amount, try to adhere to this as much as possible. Make sleep central to your life and build your life around it. That's exactly what I did with 9KM BY 9AM.

In the ten months or so since I started 9KM BY 9AM, there have been only two days when I went to bed later than 10pm and, in doing so, I upset the system. The first was staying up to watch the US Open golf, which finished in the early hours. I still got up to do my early morning walk but I felt the pain later in the day, nodding off to sleep a couple of times during the day. I also stayed up to watch a film that finished around midnight, during the Christmas break. This had a similar effect. What I should have done was sleep through, making sure I got my six and a half to seven hours. That's the plan next time this happens.

THE BENEFITS OF A GOOD NIGHT'S SLEEP

I love waking up with a fresh mouth as opposed to feeling like my mouth is like the bottom of a birdcage. This is what my mouth used to feel like in the mornings after a few drinks the night before.

An alcohol-free you is a great base on which to build the best sleeping habits. For me, improved sleep has led to more energy, more creativity, better attention, weight loss, massively reduced anxiety and stress, no feelings of depression, and there was something else... oh yes, better memory!

HOW TO GO TO BED EARLIER

Generally, it's easier to push away sleep than to advance sleep, according to sleep professor Rafael Pelayo. He says that going to bed earlier is hard to do and recommends going slowly and in small increments, adjusting no more than 15 minutes earlier every two to three days.

I didn't need to do this because I was naturally tired from all the walking. As soon as it hits 9pm, I start to fall asleep and so have to go to bed.

EARLY HOURS DICTAPHONE

According to Gary Keller, author of *The One Thing*, 'Structuring the early hours of your day is the simplest way to extraordinary results.'

Science shows that morning is the time when willpower is at its highest levels. Willpower is like a muscle – as you use it throughout the day it becomes tired but in the morning, it is at its strongest and full of energy.

The two and half hours when I am out walking are the most productive of my entire day. I use my iPhone and AirPods to make notes covering my plans for the day, ideas for my books, my client projects and anything that needs to go on a 'to do' list. An app translates my voice into words which I can edit on screen or print out on my return to the office.

The smart phone is the modern equivalent of a Dictaphone, which was popular in the 1980s to dictate messages while on the go. This reminds me of an old joke, which is probably not as funny in the 21st century as it was in the late 20th. Person 1: 'Can I borrow your Dictaphone?' Person 2: 'No, use your finger, like everyone else!' Apologies.

STEPS YOU CAN TAKE

STEP 1 – YOUR OPTIMUM LEVEL OF SLEEP

To get there, firstly work out what is the optimum number of hours you need. For an adult, it's normally between seven and nine.

To do this, go to sleep without an alarm clock and make a note of what time you fall asleep and what time you wake up. If you have to be up early for work during the week, do your test at the weekend.

STEP 2 – DOS & DON'TS

Here is a list of dos and don'ts I actioned to improve my sleep. Take a look and incorporate a few into your schedule. It could make a huge difference to your well-being.

DON'T	DO
• Drink coffee. If you do, only drink it in the morning.	• Dim the lights in your bedroom. Use a soft light to read.
• Take your phone to bed with you. Turn it off 15 minutes before you go to sleep or if you are using the alarm, put it on airplane mode.	• Make your bedroom as dark as possible. Double line curtains. If you can't black out the room, try a sleep mask.
• Sleep in a room that's too warm – it should be 10 degrees cooler than it is in the house in the daytime. Don't leave central heating or electric fires on as you'll wake up too hot in the middle of the night.	• Try earplugs if your area is noisy. • Exercise – it's good for helping you sleep. Research shows that exercising in the morning leads to more deep sleep than afternoon exercise.
• Eat too close to bedtime – this can give you heartburn.	• Meditate – it's a good way to fall asleep.
• Exercise too close to bedtime – this can wake you up.	• Get up at the same time each day, even at weekends.
• Sleep in. Once you have reached a workable bedtime and a consistent wake-up time, don't allow yourself to stray from it.	
• Drink alcohol!	

KEY LEARNINGS

• When I stopped drinking alcohol, I immediately had more energy and woke up earlier, full of life. This happens to the majority of people who stop drinking.

I think in the early days this 'Wide Awake Club' feeling is caused by a comparison your mind and body makes with the old and new you.

- Without realising it I was trading the two hours between 9.30pm and 11.30pm for the three hours between 5am and 8am the next day. Basically, I was going to bed earlier and waking up earlier the next day and getting a full six and a half to seven hours uninterrupted sleep each night.

- In the last days of my alcohol drinking life, nothing good was happening in the evening other than drinking and eating snacks, mixed with watching copious amounts of TV.

- Maximising the use of the early morning hours unlocked my life and allowed me to get fit and learn new things, as opposed to drinking and watching loads of TV, most of which I could not remember anyway!

- Once you know your optimum amount, try and sleep this every night. Try to adhere to this as much as possible. Make sleep central to your life and build your life around it.

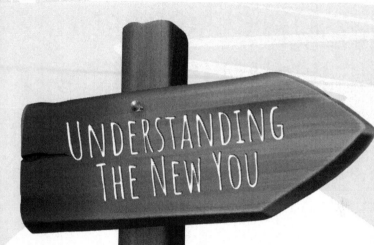

UNDERSTANDING
THE NEW YOU

THE FIRST
FEW MONTHS

UNDERSTANDING THE NEW YOU: THE FIRST FEW MONTHS

Getting deeper into the journey, I put a scaffolding structure around the house that is my body and mind. This provides an opportunity for me to live both a physically and mentally fit life. It allows me to build new, and repair and refurbish old parts of my house.

The building has many rooms:

My physical fitness – my heart, lungs, liver, muscles.

My mental well-being – the way I react, my calmness, empathy, gratitude, compassion for others.

My behaviour – my diet, habits, values, beliefs, purpose, goals.

This section of three chapters pulls together the best thinking I discovered along my journey. I have gained wisdom from ideas that have stood the test of time, including Stoicism, Buddhist teachings and the natural world around us.

I hope these thousand-year-old philosophies will help you cement the New You and show you how you can challenge yourself to do extraordinary things.

CHAPTER 19
TAKE OR CREATE A CHALLENGE

A path less travelled within my alcohol-free journey had emerged and I took it.

MY STORY

From Day One, I was feeling happier, looking years younger, starting to lose weight and had huge amounts of energy – energy that I had not experienced for many years.

By the third day of going alcohol-free, a feeling of well-being had kicked in and I felt like going for a run! This was definitely a new me. I very rarely ran and was not sure how far I could go without getting short of breath and collapsing.

I set myself an initial challenge of running 1km each day and timed myself to see how much I would improve over a month.

I used the MAPMYRIDE app to measure the time and distance and set off wearing some dusted-off trainers, tracksuit bottoms and a waterproof jacket. The first run was 1km, took 11 minutes, and was more of a 200-metre jog interspersed with a brisk walk. I know it does not sound the quickest of times, but it was something I was immensely proud of because I had crossed a barrier. I had a new belief, a new value, a new me.

By Day Four, I had ducked under 10 minutes. After one month, I recorded 1km in eight minutes, 40 seconds. I felt great. I felt alive. Running, or having a regular exercise regime, was working.

Throughout the next three months, January, February and March, I walked and cycled three times a week and was getting fitter. But there was no real plan in place, other than that I felt healthy and was going to go for a walk or a cycle ride whenever I could.

VIRTUAL CHALLENGES

At the end of March, I started a virtual walk challenge from Land's End to John O'Groats. This is a great way to exercise. Virtual walk apps track every step you walk against a real route. So, if I walked 1,000 steps around my house, this would count as 1,000 steps on the road to John O'Groats.

My sister, who lives in London, had started this virtual walk and had sent me a virtual postcard from Cornwall. She had just begun and was about 20 miles down the road. This was exactly what I needed. I called her to see if she would like me to accompany her, or put another way, race her to John O'Groats.

I'd never heard of virtual challenges, but with my new open mind and willingness to learn, I agreed to take up the challenge. For the next couple of months, we were neck and neck, walking through Cornwall, Devon, Dorset, Somerset, and the Midlands, on our way to Scotland. This gave me the walking bug – big time! Every step I took was a step closer to the goal of John O'Groats. During April and most of May, I was walking four to five kilometres a day.

At the outset of the Land's End to John O' Groats Challenge, I had allowed myself six months to complete the 1,743km distance. To hit this target, I needed to walk around 14,000 steps, or 9.5km, a day.

My step count on my *Apple Health* app was usually around 4,500 a day. In April, it jumped to over 11,000 and by May, to over 13,000. I was now checking my position daily on the virtual challenge map versus the pacemaker – a virtual marker showing where you should be in order to cross the line in the six-month time limit.

To stay on track, I needed to seriously up my game. I started to do this towards the end of May, walking early in the morning and finishing before 9am so it would not interfere with my work.

On the third day of walking 9km and finishing before 9am, the name 9KM BY 9AM came to me.

THE BIRTH OF 9KM BY 9AM

This virtual challenge walk to John O'Groats was the catalyst to 9KM BY 9AM.

I was walking along the Pilgrim's Way near to where I live in Charing, Kent, thinking to myself that I really needed to walk 15,000 steps each day. This, plus the 4,000-odd steps I would do walking around in the day, would take me up to the target to get to John O'Groats on time, or even ahead of time.

The only way I could do this was to make time for it. The best solution was to do it in the morning, as I was now waking up much earlier as a side-effect of not drinking alcohol.

Early in the morning worked well as I run a business, so if I could get the walking done before 9am then everything would fall into place.

A path less travelled within the alcohol-free journey had emerged and I took it. Little did I know then how important this one decision would be in helping to change the direction of my life. The wheels of change had been set in motion by me stopping drinking, but now a whole new force was coming into play. This was the domino effect at work.

As a child, I remember my mother always saying to me how she got up early and that, 'an hour in the morning is worth two in the day'. I think she had got that from her mum. I just remember her talking about getting things done by an early hour. So, 9KM BY 9AM was born.

This was an exciting time for me because I now had a project that I owned. I had created a vehicle to drive both my physical and mental health fitness forward. This was no longer about stopping drinking. That domino had fallen and caused a new domino to come into play that was allowing me to make big changes in my life. A plan to walk 9km every day was a trajectory that would, and did, put me on a path to fitness.

After 11 months, I had done 334 walks, pretty much every day, before 9am. It added up to 3,185kms or 1,979 miles. That's the equivalent of over 75 marathons! I hadn't set the goal of walking 75 marathons in the first 11 months. I think that if I had, I would not have been able to achieve it because it would have seemed too daunting a task. However, the daily goal to get up at 5.15am and go for a 9km walk was straightforward and achievable, and it led to a huge domino effect in my life. This is a journey goal; it is not a huge mountain to conquer but an achievable daily project.

9KM BY 9AM – THE FIRST MONTHS

MONTH	NUMBER OF WALKS	TOTAL DURATION	TOTAL DISTANCE COVERED (KMS)
May	6	14 hours 02 minutes	55.85
June	29	75 hours 37 minutes	291.39
July	29	73 hours 17 minutes	282.86
August	31	77 hours 36 minutes	293.36

September	29	74 hours 52 minutes	285.56
October	30	74 hours 38 minutes	300.14
November	29	71 hours 48 minutes	288.85
December	30	65 hours 35 minutes	286.01
January	31	68 hours 20 minutes	283.09
February	29	70 hours 53 minutes	260.62
March	31	74 hours 57 minutes	282.44
April	30	70 hours 47 minutes	275.59
Total	**334**	**812 hours 22 minutes**	**3,185.76**

Based on a marathon being 42.195kms this is the equivalent of 75.5 marathons.

STEPS – NOT THE BAND

Six months after going alcohol-free, my average daily step count was just under 20,000 steps a day, up from 4,800 per day in the last month that I was still drinking alcohol. This shows without any question of doubt the power of alcohol-free living and taking a challenge.

As far as the race to John O'Groats played out, 9KM BY 9AM had really upped my game and I pulled away from my sister, reaching the finish line in 157 days – 25 days ahead of the target of 182 days.

At the time of writing this, my average daily steps for the past year are 20,000!

9KM BY 9AM IS A WAY OF LIFE

9KM BY 9AM allows me to carry out the physical, mental and spiritual work I have set through my goals. It allows me to live my life with an open mind – to learn, to question, to live life to the full. To fulfil my purpose.

I knew there was something special about the name. It was catchy, memorable and unique. It also 'did what it said on the side of the tin', that is, walk nine kilometres before 9 o'clock in the morning.

I was committed to making this challenge a central part of who I was. Through 9KM BY 9AM, I would be able to hit all my goals because 9KM BY 9AM, by its very nature, would allow me to get physically fit. And, if I was fit in body, I would be fit in mind as the two are interlocked.

9KM BY 9AM is about doing something challenging early in the day. For me, it is walking 9km. For others, it could be walking 1km, running 3km, cycling 15km, writing a song, reading a book, painting a landscape – everyone is different.

The 9KM BY 9AM social media channels are a fly-on-the-wall view into alcohol-free living journeys of all who post there. My plan from the outset was to provide an inspiration to others so they can create their own challenges on their pathway or journey.

MENTAL CHALLENGE

9KM BY 9AM is not just physical. It's about the ideas, the thoughts, the creativity, and the time to think that I have on the walks. Most of the ideas in this book came to me when I am out walking early, learning new things through listening to podcasts and audio books, and reflecting on ideas I heard the day before.

I think it's important to become not just a student of alcohol-free living, but a student of life. By that, I mean learn everything you can – from books, the internet and any other sources. *9KM BY 9AM* has allowed me to do this and is part of the secret – but not the whole secret.

WHAT I LEARNT

I am so grateful that I developed the challenge mentality that stopping drinking allowed me to nurture. This challenge mentality has helped me to live my life to the full and feel the best I have felt, both mentally and physically, since I was in my twenties – over 25 years ago!

MINDFULNESS ON THE MOVE

The early morning walks offered me an ideal opportunity to practise mindfulness. In fact, I do all my meditations while on the move. It works for me, so it could work for you too. There is a whole chapter on mindfulness but I'll just touch briefly here on what I do each day on the walks.

In the early days, when I was learning how to meditate and reach a state of mindfulness, I listened to guided meditations, mainly from Tara Brach. Initially, I was learning how to focus through breathing to clear my mind and find the space between my thoughts where I knew I could be present.

The beauty of walking in the countryside and parks is that you are close to nature, and it is easier to switch off and become present with what is around you, particularly very early in the morning when there are less distractions. In fact, the only distractions are the things you want to be aware of, such as the birds singing, the sunrise, the movement of the clouds, the sound of the wind in the trees, the rain falling on your jacket, the footsteps of your dog, the rustling of the leaves.

It's amazing how much time you have to yourself – to think, to listen, to learn, to increase your wisdom, to take on new concepts, to change your beliefs.

PUSHING MYSELF

As I move well into my second year of alcohol-free living, the challenges I am setting myself are getting bigger and more challenging.

For 2022, I set myself a number of personal challenges and also ones that involve my nearest and dearest.

These include a *Mountain A Month Challenge* – walking up at least one mountain each month. The first was Pen y Fan, the highest mountain in South Wales at 886 metres, which I completed a few days ago. The experience was one I will never forget. I was lucky to do it with my son and it was great to achieve something together. At one point, I was crawling on my hands and knees near the summit because the wind was so strong. A nightmare at the time but great memories now.

One year ago, I wouldn't have been able to do this. But now I can and I did. Nothing is impossible. This is something I have learnt since going alcohol-free.

Life is getting better, with richer content. My wife and I are planning to tour the UK, taking the *9KM BY 9AM* Challenge around Britain. We plan to buy a camper van, park in different spots and use this as the base camp for the start of several walks in different parts of the country.

These new challenges feel like a natural progression. The challenges are getting more exciting. I am starting to live my life to the full.

STEPS YOU CAN TAKE

STEP 1 – CHOOSE A CHALLENGE

9KM BY 9AM was my main challenge; it is the way I do it. The scaffolding I put around myself. What works for me might work for you. But you have to figure your own way through it. You have to want it and to live it if you are going to achieve it.

There is no one single way. Everyone is different and everyone has a different path. My challenges are part of my journey but hopefully you can see something in these that is relevant to you and your view of the world. I can give you pointers and guides, but it's ultimately down to you. Steps 2 to 6 below are a few things you could do.

STEP 2 – TRY A 9KM BY 9AM WALK

To walk 9km, you need to be out of bed by 5.30am at the latest. It takes me 20 minutes to wash and dress, and just over two hours and 10 minutes to walk the distance at a moderate pace, including making a daily video and taking photographs. Then it takes roughly 45 minutes to change, shower and dress and have breakfast when I arrive back home. If I am not starting the walk from my house and need to drive somewhere, I get up earlier. That's why *8KM BY 8AM* was never an option!

Some people express concerns about getting up so early each day. Once I went alcohol-free, I soon realised that the mornings are the best time of the day. I naturally wake up at 5am, wide-eyed and ready for the day ahead because I don't drink alcohol.

If you do not fancy walking, then replace it with a run, cycling, rowing, writing, painting or whatever else appeals to you.

STEP 3 – TAKE A VIRTUAL CHALLENGE

There are quite a few virtual walk apps to choose from. I use the *Conqueror* app, which has a wide selection of routes and also plants a real tree for every 20% of a challenge completed – or five trees per challenge.

Taking a challenge gave me something to look forward to. It gave me a purpose and helped drive my daily step numbers and general fitness in the right direction. You can take a challenge by yourself and at your own pace. I did the first one with/against my sister but you're never really alone because there are lots of other 'real' people you see on the virtual road.

The walks do have a bit of an addictive side to them, but that's a good thing because you're getting fitter. As soon as I completed the 1,000-mile plus walk to John O'Groats, I immediately started my second challenge – the walk from Chicago to LA, via the famous Route 66, which I am currently on. At 2,280 miles, this is more than twice the distance of Land's End to John O'Groats. I have set myself a year to do it and I am currently 87% of the way there after 257 days, so should finish it in nine and a half months!

If the thought of walking long distances scares you, there are lots of shorter routes: Berlin Wall 30 miles (48.3km); Easter Island 38 miles (61.1km); Mount Everest 39.9 miles (64.2km); or you can set your own challenge route.

STEP 4 – STEP COUNTS

Set yourself a steps count goal. Two years ago, I was happy with 5,000 steps a day and 10,000 was a big day. Now I am not happy until I have done at least 17,500 and 30,000 is a big day. Raise your bar. It will have massive effects on every aspect of your life.

STEP 5 – GET CREATIVE

Challenges do not have to be physical. There are loads of different things you can do. I decided I wanted to learn the piano. Here are a few suggestions:

Learn to play a musical instrument. It is amazing how present you become when learning an instrument. You have to focus, and this sends you into a form of trance. Hours can pass in what seems like minutes because you become so engrossed. There are beginner and advanced courses for almost all instruments – why not give one a go? Do you fancy learning guitar, ukulele, banjo, piano, saxophone or recorder?

Unleash the artist within you. Learn to draw, paint, sculpt. Learn to write songs, poetry, stories, books. Give it a go.

For most of these, all you need is a pencil and a blank piece of paper. There are also hundreds of thousands of free 'how to do it' videos on the web.

I heard someone say that learning is like jumping into a pit full of muddy, gloriously messy knowledge. It's OK to get messy and to get things wrong because this is the best way to learn. It's where the fun lives. It's tempting to sit on the side-lines, and never fail or get anything wrong, but this is not where the fun lives. You can't learn unless you get down and dirty at some point.

STEP 6 – FOREST BATHING

Lastly, one of the things I love most about early morning walks is the Japanese practice of shinrin-yoku. In Japanese, *shinrin* means 'forest' and *yoku* means 'bath'. So shinrin-yoku means bathing in the forest atmosphere, by taking in the forest through the senses. It is simply being in nature, connecting with it through the senses of sight, hearing, taste, smell and touch. Shinrin-yoku is like a bridge. By opening our senses, it bridges the gap between you and the natural world.

I do this more so in the summer months. Find a quiet place in a wood where you can sit on the floor and let the forest in. Savour the sounds, smells, sights, touch and even the taste of nature. Listen to the wind brush through the leaves, smell the morning mist, see the light break through the branches, touch the bark of a tree and taste running water from a stream.

A 30-minute forest bath once or twice a week will help you slow down. It will bring you into the present moment and de-stress and relax you.

KEY LEARNINGS

- Stopping drinking allows you to nurture a challenge mentality that will help you live your life to the full.

- A daily challenge is a vehicle to drive forward both your physical and mental health fitness forward. It can put you on a trajectory that will change your life.

- Don't just become a student of alcohol-free living but a student of life. Learn everything you can, from books, the internet and any other sources.

- Set yourself personal challenges that involve your nearest and dearest. Use them to build connections.

- Do it now, do it right now. Take the challenge. Don't sit on the side-lines and worry about failing or getting stuff wrong.

CHAPTER 20
THROW OUT YOUR DIET BOOKS – JUST STOP DRINKING

By stopping drinking, I was consuming less calories from liquid refreshment and burning more through my new-found energy and love of walking.

MY STORY

I started writing this chapter thinking I had discovered some new, fantastic diet that would make me millions. But the reality is that it's not really a diet. It's just me following my journey goals every day, which are: don't drink alcohol; get up between 5am and 5.30am and go for a 9km walk; and meditate for 15 minutes.

My new 'typical' day schedule and activities meant I was eating in a ten-hour window. I was not eating for 14 or 15 hours each day, effectively a 10/14 or 9/15 intermittent-fasting diet. I was on a diet without knowing I was on a diet and that, I believe, made all the difference as there was absolutely no pressure to diet.

I'd lost just over a stone in weight in the first six months of the alcohol-free journey, going from 17 stone 11lbs (112kg) to 16 stone 8lb (105kg), just by cutting out ALL alcohol and the snacks that went with that habit. My focus in the early days was beating alcohol – nothing else.

As I progressed on the journey, I became more aware that I had to up my game physically and exercise more. I started to become more aware of what I was eating, driven by the fact that I had stopped drinking and by the well-being doors that were opening up every day for me. I just wanted to be healthier; it was becoming a self-fulfilling prophecy.

The real magic, in the form of significant weight loss, started to happen from six months onwards, after I started the 9km walks, coupled with the 10/14 diet I did not realise I was on. In four months, I was 15 stone (95kg) and by 8 months, 14 stone (88kg). In 14 months, I had lost 3 stone 11lbs (24kg) and am continuing to lose weight, just by living the AF lifestyle.

ME & DIETS

Like most men in their 50s, I'd never openly talked about my diet. The more I delved into my past, the more I realised that I'd played around with loads of diets from the fringes, throughout my life.

The one that stands out the most and showed the most immediate results was the Atkins Diet, which I did in the early '90s. I lost over a stone in two weeks of just eating protein and fat. I had bad breath as a result, but the pounds fell off. As with all diets I tried, however, from that point onwards, the pounds crept back on. Within a month or two, I was back where I started.

I'd also tried counting calories with *Weight Watchers* in my 40s. This worked for a while, but I found myself forgoing food so that I could still have a bottle of wine each night!

Towards the end of my drinking career, I used a few diet apps. The one that stands out was *Lose It!*, recommended to me by a doctor friend. Basically, you input all the food and drink you consume into the app, which tracks your calorie intake and gives you a daily calories allowance based on your target weight loss. This is also linked to health apps and step count so you can build up food allowance by burning calories.

It is a really good way to become aware of what you are eating and the calorie content of foods. However, I started to work it so I could still drink a bottle of wine a day and stay on the diet. I did this by skipping snacks and going for walks to build up my calories burnt. This is how the mind of someone who likes a bottle of wine each night works!

Looking back on it, these diets were doomed to fail because they were not changing my lifestyle; they were just fads to me. There was no long-term goal. And through all these diets, I never once stopped drinking alcohol. I simply built it into the diet.

Any of these diets could have worked if I had truly believed in them, but I did not.

I am not saying that you can't lose weight while you drink alcohol but, for me, alcohol was a root cause of putting on weight and was the central part of an altogether unhealthy lifestyle. There are so many calories in alcohol but it does not stop there. Once you have had a few drinks, you get more relaxed about eating junk food, like salty snacks and fried meals.

By my early 50s, I was drinking roughly half a bottle of spirits (ABV 40%), seven bottles of wine (ABV 12.5%) and six pints of beer (ABV 5%) each week. That's around 6,500 calories a week in alcohol alone. That's more than two and half days' worth of my recommended food allowance.

DAILY FOOD & EXERCISE SCHEDULE

My daily schedule now is, roughly:

5am	wake up naturally
5.30am to 8.30am	exercise: 9KM BY 9AM walk
8.30am to 9am	eat breakfast
12pm to 1pm	eat lunch
6pm to 6.30pm	eat dinner
9pm to 10pm	go to bed/go to sleep

Plus two or three High Intensity Training (HIT) sessions throughout the day. Five to ten minutes of sit ups, press ups and weights.

DAILY FOOD & DRINK

	FOOD	DRINK
BREAKFAST	Weekdays Bowl containing banana, muesli, bran flakes, porridge oats, honey, soya milk Weekends 3 x pieces of toast with butter and marmalade	Tea – 2 x mugs every morning
LUNCH	Sandwich – for example, cheese and salad Or omelette Or something vegan	Tea – 1 x mug every lunchtime

DINNER	Vegetarian meal – for example, risotto, cauliflower cheese, fajitas, Greek-style kebabs, Thai curry, pasta, vegan pie	Water or squash or AF Beer
SNACKS	Homemade cake Apples Homemade biscuits – normally with tea	Tea with soya milk – 1 x litre tea throughout day Coffee – once a week on Saturday ½ litre of water as soon as I get up, daily ½ litre water on 9KM BY 9AM walk, daily
THINGS I SHOULD NOT EAT A LOT OF	Chips – once a week Pizza – once a week Chocolate bars – one a week Salted peanuts – once a fortnight	

I'm eating around 2,500 to 3,000 calories a day and I'm burning around 1,000 calories each morning on the 9KM BY 9AM walk, plus around 2,500 calories in energy needed to live throughout the day. The net effect is that I'm burning more than I'm consuming.

The important thing here is I do not look at this as a diet. It's just what I do. I'm never hungry. I eat great food and I exercise throughout the day.

On the 9KM BY 9AM walks, my heart rate is on average around 100 to 120 beats per minute, for at least two and a half hours. So, I am getting a very long, low-aerobic workout.

MEAT FREE

Just over a year after stopping drinking alcohol, I decided to stop eating meat. As I write this, I am coming up to four months meat free. I initially thought I'd do a month to try it out, but I am really enjoying it on several levels.

In part, I have been heavily influenced by my family. My wife has been a vegetarian most of her life. My elder daughter is a vegan and my younger daughter a vegetarian. My son, who has left home for university, is the only one in our family of five who eats meat. Given this, I was eating three or four vegetarian evening meals a week. My meat intake was chicken twice a week and ham in sandwiches at lunchtime a couple of times a week, plus bacon for breakfast on the weekend. I rarely ate fish because my wife is allergic to it and I ate steak three or four times a year.

So, the transition to meat free was not a big physical bridge but more a psychological one.

On a personal level, I was feeling healthier and more conscious about my body and what food I was eating. This was supported by the fact that it's hard to ignore the suffering that animals go through *en route* to the plate. Topping this off, is the difference that stopping eating meat would make to global warming if enough people stopped. I still eat some dairy, mainly cheese, and wear leather shoes so I suppose I could be seen as being a bit hypocritical!

One hundred or so days into meat-free living, I do feel healthier. It's hard to explain until you cross the bridge, but I'm enjoying the huge range of plant-based foods now readily available in supermarkets and restaurants, and they just feel like the healthier option.

At the end of the day, it's each to their own. If you like meat, go on eating it. These are just my views and it makes me happy to live this way.

THE GYM

After the first few months of stopping drinking, I decided to turn our garden summer house into a gym. 'Drinking me' would never have done this. Today, I am the proud owner of my own gym, with cycle workout station, weights and punch bag, which I use daily.

Throughout my adult life, I have had several gym memberships. I had joined these gyms because I felt that I needed to get fit. These were mostly affairs that started in January as daily workouts and ended up as a very expensive sauna once a month by the spring!

I also had access to a gym when I lived in Singapore. The apartment I rented was part of a condo that came with a shared swimming pool, bowling green, tennis courts and a gym. When I was looking for apartments, one of the main selling points were the amenities. As with my gym memberships, this started off well, with maybe three or four visits to my condo gym, but within three weeks, it was a place I never went to again.

The only exception to this rule was a membership I took out to a gym near our village in Kent. I had this for around five years and did use it actively in my 30s. Without a doubt, I was inspired by my desire to play an active part in the lives of our three young children. I had a real 'Why' inspiring me to make a real change. This is so true for any major change you make to your health lifestyle. You have got to really want to do it, and to do it successfully, you need a solid reason or 'Why'.

I recently moved a couple of weights and an exercise ball next to the desk in my office. Every hour or so, I get up and pump some iron and do a few press-ups and sit-ups. When it gets warmer, I'll go into the garden and hit the punchbag, which is hanging up outside.

WHAT I LEARNT

I believe I would not have lost weight if I kept on drinking.

That's it – throw out the diet books! All you need to do is stop drinking alcohol and the rest will take care of itself. That's what happened to me.

In the 15 months since I stopped drinking alcohol, I have not restricted what I eat or stopped eating types of food because I HAD to or NEEDED to. Any changes I have made I have done because I WANTED to and that is the magical difference.

I used to eat lots of crisps, biscuits, chocolate bars. But now I don't. The reason is that I don't want to. Just like I don't want to jump out of an upstairs window. I have no desire to.

Being AF means no hangovers, and no hangovers mean no cravings for fried food and all the other junk I would eat to try and feel normal again. It also means a decimation of the amount of salty snacks I threw down my neck. Yes, I still love the odd salted peanut but on nothing like the scale I used to.

The main thing about being alcohol-free is that you start to question everything about your well-being – how much you exercise; what you eat; what you drink; how much you sleep.

STEPS YOU CAN TAKE

STEP 1 – STOP DRINKING ALCOHOL

Stop drinking alcohol for three months and see what happens to you.

Ask yourself these questions after three months alcohol-free.

- Am I eating healthier food because I want to?

- Am I exercising more because I want to?
- Am I sleeping better?
- Do I have more energy?
- Am I feeling fitter?
- Is there a noticeable increase in my well-being?
- Have I lost weight?

The answer should be yes for everything. It was for me.

KEY LEARNINGS

- For any major change you make to your health lifestyle – you have got to really want to do it and to do it successfully you need a solid reason or 'Why'.

- When you stop drinking, well-being doors will start to open for you every day.

- By stopping drinking, you consume less calories from liquid refreshment and burn more through new-found energy.

- Diets are doomed to fail if you do not build them into your lifestyle. They are then just fads. There has to be a long-term goal. If 'stopping drinking alcohol' becomes your long-term goal, you will more than likely start to lose weight.

- Being AF means no hangovers, and no hangovers mean less cravings for fried food and all the other junk you eat to try and feel normal again. It also means a decimation of the amount of salty snacks you'll consume.

CHAPTER 21
BECOME A STUDENT OF PHILOSOPHY

'Under the floor of some poor man's house lies a treasure.
But because he does not know of its existence, he does not
think he is rich. Similarly, inside one man's mind lies truth
itself, firm and unfading. Yet because beings see it not,
they experience a constant stream of misery. The treasure
of truth lies within the house of the mind.'
Maitreya Buddha

MY STORY

I absolutely love this quote. It was one of the first things
I read from a book on Buddhist teachings. It was a WOW
moment for me. A realisation that the answer to all my life's
problems is within me. True happiness and contentment
are not a bigger house or a faster car, or a holiday on a
tropical island. The treasure of true happiness had been
sitting in my mind since birth. I just did not know where
to look.

With the wisdom gained through thousand-year-old
Eastern and Western philosophies, together with a new-
found appreciation of the natural world around me, I was
propelled along my alcohol-free pathway. I was gaining a
clearer understanding of who I am; how the human mind

works; a more balanced view of my life; and the drive to challenge myself to do extraordinary things.

THE MEANING OF MY LIFE

Wisdom and learning, and using the knowledge I gain to give back, are a central part of my core values.

The internal superpower I unleashed by becoming alcohol-free created a huge thirst to learn more about science, religion, philosophy, spiritualism. In fact, to learn about anything that would improve my well-being and my understanding of who I am, why I'm here and the meaning of life.

When I was drinking, I never really gave the meaning of my life a great deal of thought, mainly because I was stuck on the hamster wheel, locked into the *Groundhog Day* existence, with a few 'relaxing' drinks to look forward to every night!

I simply did not have time, as this was earmarked, or dog-eared, for drinking. And drinking alcohol makes you non-present.

Being alcohol-free means that I now have an abundance of time to read and practise what I learn. It helps improve my well-being and allows me to break through the glass ceiling that keeps so many on the alcohol-living wheel all their lives.

There are several philosophies that stood out. I explain the thoughts within those philosophies that made a real difference to me.

STOICISM

It was my 18-year-old son who initially introduced me to Stoicism. Of course, I had heard of it, but I had never had the time to let it in to do its magic.

Stoicism dates back to Ancient Greek and Roman times but is as relevant today as it was then. Famous Stoic writers include Seneca and Epictetus. Probably the most famous is the Roman Emperor Marcus Aurelius, whose personal journal called *Meditations* is, in my opinion, one of the most powerful books ever written.

I signed up to Ryan Holiday's *Daily Stoic* channel, with its Stoic thought of the day email, plus access to the daily podcast with interviews with Stoic thinkers. I bought a few of Ryan's books, as well as Marcus Aurelius' *Meditations* and submerged myself in Stoicism.

The aim of Stoicism is to lead a good life and stay resilient in tough times. At its core, are four virtues, namely: Wisdom, Justice, Temperance and Courage. Every situation, every moment, is an opportunity to exemplify these forms of human excellence. There is no challenge or problem so big that it does not call for wisdom, justice, temperance and/ or courage.

I even bought a coin engraved with these virtues, plus several Stoic principles, which I carry around with me. I started to live my life by these principles and still do today. They are: The Obstacle Is The Way; Remember That You Die; Ego Is The Enemy; Be Grateful For What You Have; and Love Your Fate.

Stoics say we don't control the world around us, but we do control how we respond. It's not what happens to you – it's the way you react that matters. Life throws 'stuff' at you. This 'stuff' is a constant test and the way we respond should be through one of the four Stoic virtues.

BUDDHISM

The world would be a much safer, better and nicer place if Buddhist teachings became more widespread and accepted in Western society. There is a huge stereotype of all Buddhists being monks in orange gowns. That's the same as thinking all Christians are priests. The reality is that Buddhism has over 500 million followers around the world and is a way of life as well as a religion. I learned so much from its teachings and implore you to drop your guard and look at these philosophies as a good way to live your life and care for all living beings and our planet. Mindfulness is a central part of Buddhism. Learning meditations and mindfulness practice based on Buddhist teaching is a great way to understand how your mind works. This can help to overcome desires for things like alcohol.

BE AWARE OF YOUR INTENTIONS

A teaching that jumped out at me the first time I read it, is the Buddhist teaching on the 'Power of Intention'. It says that our entire life arises out of the spirit of intention. From intention springs the deed. From deeds spring the habits. From the habits grow the character. From the character develops the destiny. So, what we intend to do shapes who we are.

Neuroscience shows that the neurons in our brains fire together and wire together. This means that the more you do something, the more it becomes a normal and accepted thing for you to do.

Depending on your intention, this can be good or bad news for you. Henry Ford's famous saying sums this up beautifully: 'Whether you think you can, or you think you can't, you're right'. This is simply self-fulfilling prophecy. If you tell yourself something, or others start telling you: 'You are this' or 'You do this', you will start to believe it. If you keep telling yourself it, you will do it and you'll become it. It will become your destiny. So, be careful of your intentions and what you wish for.

This holds for everything. If you intend to drink alcohol every day, it will soon become your destiny. If you eat well and work out every day, you will become fit.

D.H. Lawrence says, 'Men are not free when they're doing just what they like. Men are only free when they're doing what the deepest self likes.' Getting down to this deepest self takes some diving.

According to psychologist Tara Brach, there are many ways to understand your deepest intentions, including the 'Wisdom of Impermanence'. This basically means you only learn when something bad happens to you and triggers you to question who you are. I started questioning my relationship with alcohol when I realised the enormous bad effects it was having on my health, my relationships and my life expectancy. This made me question my intentions and what I wanted out of my life.

Another way is to just start questioning. Step outside yourself and ask yourself, 'What are my intentions?' In short, you need to shift from an ego intention to an aspirational intention and by that, I mean ask yourself, 'What do I aspire to be? What is my purpose?'

Tara Brach says, all we have is the present moment, the people around us, and our connections. These are the things that matter. Let these guide your intentions and let your heart be your compass.

THE PARABLE OF THE SECOND ARROW

Another great teaching that I practise a lot is the parable of the second arrow. This is easy to do. It's so simple, yet so powerful. The teaching says there are two arrows for every event that happens to you. The first arrow is the event itself. It's what happens. It could be: someone was horrible to you; you had an accident; you broke up with your partner; you stopped drinking. The second arrow is how you react to the first arrow. Remember that every single thought you think comes from within you. No one else is thinking it. Just you. Whether it's fear of missing out, anxiety, craving or grasping, the thought comes from within you. So, when I craved a drink, I viewed this as a second arrow. The more you realise that this second arrow is on its way, the better the chance you have of dealing with it, being ready for it and watching it whizz by.

JAPANESE PHILOSOPHY

I read lots of Japanese philosophy. I did not plan to do this. I just fell into it and the more I discovered, the bigger my appetite became for it.

WABI SABI

One of the many philosophies I have taken on board is the Japanese aesthetic of Wabi Sabi. Loosely translated, 'wabi' is simplicity, whether elegant or rustic, and 'sabi' means the beauty of age and wear. It's about seeing the perfection in imperfection and recognising that all things are impermanent. It teaches you not to pile pressure on yourself in the pursuit of perfection. Wabi Sabi is a great way to put everything in perspective because perfection is a delusion and everything is perfectly imperfect!

Wabi Sabi also explains 'learning' as never being complete. There is no complete or perfect 'learning' and we should approach it with that in mind. When you start to learn something new, like living an alcohol-free life, Wabi Sabi says you should embark on your journey with the understanding that there isn't a final destination. 'Learning' never ends. It also never helps to compare yourself to others further along the path of 'learning', as well as those way behind. You should focus only on your individual journey.

SEKKI & KO

As I walked 9km each morning as part of 9KM BY 9AM, I started to pay more attention to the natural world around me and the changes that were happening. Around the same time, I also discovered through a podcast I was listening to, that the Japanese have names for 24 short seasons called *sekki* and 72 micro seasons, known as *kō*.

These seasons are designed to make us better understand our connection with nature. By being aware of the finer changes in the environment, we can learn to be more present and in rhythm with the outside world. They have names like '*Awakening of hibernated insects*', '*First peach* blossoms', 'Worms surface', 'Cool winds blow' and 'Mist starts to hover'.

By paying attention to nature, I began to notice a whole world of magic. I started to live in the now, by sensing the small changes in the outside world as they happened.

These shorter seasons enable you to learn to read slight changes in the natural world and become more sensitive to your own rhythms. They show you the transient nature of everything. Flowers blossom and wilt; insects die; snow melts. This reminds us of our own impermanence and tells you that you must focus on what really matters now, before it's too late.

HAPPY FOR NO REASON

After taking on board these philosophies and ideas, I started to feel 'happiness' without having to tie it to something. I am just happy and content because I understand who I am and what my purpose is. Happiness was once just linked to watching a great movie, going on holiday, buying a new guitar or playing sport. I am still happy when things like that happen, but I now have a deeper happiness and contentment.

I heard a metaphor recently about indigo cloth and its unique, deep, rich blue colour. It takes some time for the cloth to get to that colour. When a white cloth is first dipped into the indigo dye, it comes out blue but then quickly fades to off-white. It's rinsed then dipped again. Once again, it fades quickly but holds a bit more colour this time. Only after many rounds of dipping does the colour of the cloth finally deepen to have that characteristic rich hue. In the same way, every moment I dipped into philosophy my inner happiness became richer and more cemented.

It's not about material things. It's nice to have a new guitar or go to a new restaurant, but these are just things. I believe happiness is driven by relationships and connections with others. I am most happy when I'm laughing with my wife, my children, my mother, my friends, my dog, my cat. Just being with them in the moment is true happiness.

But the connection does not stop there! Happiness is also driven by connecting with the environment, with what's around you: sunrises, sunsets, trees, country lanes, mountains, beaches, the sea, waves, the moon, the stars. Just being aware that these things are there is amazing and at the heart of feeling contentment. Also, connecting with wisdom, with all the great creations and ideas that have gone before – books, plays, films, music.

WHAT I LEARNT

Philosophy helps me understand my purpose. It helps me become more present and to be there for the ones I love. It helps me find true happiness and contentment.

Like all the philosophies I touch on here, it is impossible to do them full justice in a few pages. I have set out below the key points I learnt, which I think are worth sharing. But this is just a start. Please see sources for further reading.

STOICISM

THE OBSTACLE IS THE WAY: This is pretty much at the heart of why I was able to become alcohol-free and change my life. The pandemic was a major obstacle for all of us who lived through it. I was lucky enough, through this simple Stoic teaching, to turn it into a positive. Marcus Aurelius says, 'The impediment to action advances action. What stands in the way becomes the way.' A Stoic finds a way to turn every negative into a positive. We always have the opportunity to practise virtue, to use the situation to become our best selves. The things that test us make us who we are. I used the pandemic as an opportunity to rethink my life and to look at what was not working. I identified my relationship with alcohol as the root of my problems and the rest is history.

MEMENTO MORI or 'Remember that you die': This is not morbid; in fact, it is 100% positive. Our time on this planet is precious, so if you want to achieve a goal of getting healthier, starting a business, going alcohol-free, or whatever it is that drives you, then don't put it off. DO IT NOW because you might be dead tomorrow! Treat your time as a gift and do not waste it. One of the biggest wastes of time I can think of is drinking. I knew I had to stop drinking. According to Stoicism, the time is now, so I acted upon this.

EGO IS THE ENEMY: The Stoics say, 'The greatest foe is your own ego.' It is important to be humble when ambitious, gracious when successful and resilient when you fail. Ego is the belief that you are better than, and more entitled than, everyone else. It's the inner voice telling you what to do. Whatever you do in life, ego is the enemy every step of the way. This is also the title of a great book by Ryan Holiday.

PREMEDITATIO MALORUM: No, I did not study Latin at school. What this means is 'the premeditation of evils'. Appreciate and be grateful for what you have. Imagine that everything that can go wrong will go wrong. By doing that, you are prepared for the worst-case scenario. If it ever happens, it won't be as big a problem as it would have been if you were not prepared! Make sense? The best way to do this is to try and understand what your life would be like if you did not have family, friends, pets, hot showers, a roof over your head, and so on. You should not take this wealth for granted. Seneca, says, 'What is quite unlooked for is more crushing in its effect and unexpectedness adds to the weight of a disaster. With anticipation, we create time to raise defences or even avoid them entirely – death, illness, divorce.'

AMOR FATI: This literally means 'love of one's fate'. It's a mindset making the best of anything that happens. Marcus Aurelius says, 'A blazing fire makes flames and brightness out of everything that is thrown into it. Embrace everything and be better for it.' Quite like the saying, 'If it does not kill you, it will make you stronger.'

SYMPATHEUM: This is the belief that there is mutual interdependence among everything in the universe – we are all one. It is an invite to take a step back, zoom out, and see life from a higher vantage point. This can turn daily worries of anxiety to absurdness. Edgar Mitchell, on Apollo 14, said, 'In outer space you develop an instant global consciousness, a people orientation, an intense dissatisfaction with the state of the world and a compulsion to do something about it.'

BUDDHIST TEACHINGS

Buddhism was founded roughly 2,500 years ago by Siddhartha Gautama, a noble person, who came to be known as The Buddha. Gautama was born to a privileged ruling family and lived a life unaware of any form of suffering, shielded by palace life. One day, he went outside the palace and encountered, for the first time, old age, sickness and death. Driven by this, at age 29, he left the comforts and power of his royal life, including his wife and son, and travelled for six years. At age 35, Siddhartha had 'The Great Awakening' to the truth about existence. While sitting under a Bodhi tree, he became enlightened. For the next 45 years, he taught the path to enlightenment.

FOUR NOBLE TRUTHS

The Buddha's first teaching, or sermon, was the Four Noble Truths. These give Buddhists the opportunity to examine and reflect upon why they are suffering in life, and how they may attempt to overcome the Three Poisons, which are at the root of all suffering: Hate, Greed and Ignorance.

It is worth noting here that any addiction or bad habit is caused by one or more of these poisons, so you can see that the teachings set out a pathway to overcome these problems.

First Truth – Dukkha. Suffering. This states that everything leads to suffering and therefore un-satisfactoriness. To overcome suffering, a Buddhist may meditate more, in order to attempt to spiritually overcome the Three Poisons. In addition, they may become more charitable, as this will help them to overcome suffering, by helping with the root cause of their pain.

Second Truth – Samudaya. Origin of Suffering. This truth is related to the cause of suffering, which is based on craving and desire.

The Buddha taught that nothing is permanent and that everything is impermanent. Therefore, people should avoid getting attached to things as eventually everything will change. People suffer when they crave and when they get attached to people and objects.

The Three Poisons only help to deepen people's desire for craving. The Buddha taught that people don't understand their cravings. He said that people get stuck in the cycle of samsara (very much like running on a hamster wheel) and, therefore, cannot reach enlightenment or find meaning in their lives.

Third Truth – Nirodha. End of Suffering. The good news is suffering can be ended. This can be obtained through the right effort and through the right actions. Buddhists engage in meditation to end cravings and become more aware of who they are.

Fourth Truth – Magga. Path of the End of Suffering. Known as the Eightfold Path, Buddhists believe this is the way to wisdom and the mental training they need to achieve the way of morality. Buddhists believe it is the 'cure' that was given by The Buddha for suffering. It provides them with the ideal way to live and can lead to enlightenment. The eight paths are having the right: View, Intention, Speech, Action, Livelihood, Effort, Concentration, and Mindfulness.

STEPS YOU CAN TAKE

This all worked for me. It might work for you.

STEP 1 – DIVE IN

There is a whole wealth of books and articles on philosophy. Search introductions to Stoicism, Buddhism, Japanese Philosophy on *Google*.

STEP 2 – SEE YOUR OWN 72 SEASONS

Go for a walk. Try and get out at least once a day. Look at the world through the philosophies you are reading. What changes can you see on your walk? Notice the flowers starting to bloom, the leaves falling off trees, the first frost. By doing this, you are living in the now.

STEP 3 – STOICISM

Make a list of the important things in your life and imagine what it would be like if they disappeared tomorrow. What would you really miss?

Subscribe to *The Daily Stoic* – receive a daily email with a Stoic thought for the day.

STEP 4 – BUDDHISM

I recommend reading a good introductory book like *Buddhism for Dummies*. It has all the main thinking in one place and gives you a grounded background. If you want to go further and learn more this is a perfect start point.

STEP 5 – MINDFULNESS OF INTENTION

Practice the mindfulness of intention. When you become aware of intention before you act, you're able to make wise choices that lead you to clarity, well-being, and harmony.

Without awareness of intention, you can easily end up reacting, living on autopilot, or mindlessly following old habits. Observing your mind closely, you'll see that intention precedes every action.

KEY LEARNINGS

- The internal superpower that is unleashed by becoming alcohol-free creates a huge appetite and thirst to learn more about science, religion, philosophy, and spiritualism.

- The aim of Stoicism is to lead a good life and stay resilient in tough times. At its core are four virtues, namely: Wisdom, Justice, Temperance, and Courage.

- Stoics say we don't control the world around us, but we do control how we respond. It's not what happens to you; it's the way you react that matters.

- Buddhism has over 500 million followers around the world and is a way of life as well as a religion. Buddhism says that our entire life arises out of the spirit of intention. From intention springs the deed. From deeds spring the habits. From the habits grow the character. From the character develops the destiny.

- Wabi Sabi is a great way to put everything in perspective because perfection is a delusion and everything is perfectly imperfect!

- Philosophy helps me understand my purpose. It helps me become more present and to be there for the ones I love. It helps me find true happiness and contentment.

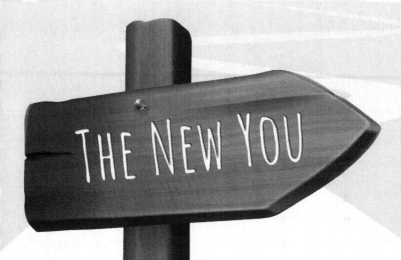

BEYOND
90 DAYS

THE NEW YOU: BEYOND 90 DAYS

Top class 100-metre sprinters say they run the first 50 metres with their legs and the next with their minds.

Similarly, once you have passed the 90-day mark, you are flying, and being alcohol-free becomes part of you.

This section looks at the small steps you can take each day to keep you on your trajectory, and how to deal with the reactions of others to your new-found love of life.

I also explore one of the hottest topics almost everyone who takes the alcohol free path asks – is it possible to moderate?

And last but not least, some tips on how to stay 'on the wagon'.

CHAPTER 22
THE MIRAGE OF MODERATION

The 'big' question for some people who recognise that they are not fully in control of their relationship with alcohol is: 'Is it possible to moderate my alcohol consumption?'

MY STORY

My answer is simply this: The ability to moderate alcohol consumption for those that have had or have issues with alcohol control is a delusion, and part of the alcohol narrative and indoctrination. I call this the 'Mirage of Moderation'. Once you realise that alcohol is poison and not good for your well-being, why on earth would you want to try and manage the amount of poison you consume? Don't drink poison. That's true control.

The fact that people discuss moderation means they realise alcohol is not good for them. They would like to restrict the amount they consume so that they can live a healthy life, totally in control of their habit.

When I drank alcohol, I could not moderate to a level I thought was good for my health. I just drank whenever I felt the urge – and that was every day.

If I had tried to be a Friday and Saturday nights-only drinker, I would have put myself through psychological torture from Sunday to Thursday. For me, alcohol was an all-or-nothing drug. In the 36 years I was a drinker, the longest I went without drinking was six days. I think I managed five days on three occasions, and a handful of three days. What I remember about these heroic ventures was that I thought about booze almost every second of the day. If that's what moderation is, then you can keep it!

I asked myself this question: Is an ex-heroin addict in control of their heroin habit if they dabble once a week, or just on their birthday or special occasions? It would be very hard to argue the case for yes.

In the early days of the alcohol-free journey, I would often think about going back to the booze and just having one glass of wine, a couple of times a week. But I knew that was just my inner voice calling me back.

I contemplated moderating for the first seven months into my journey. After that, the voice that says, 'When you get to one year, you could probably have a couple of drinks,' simply went away. I never entertained the idea of moderation again.

Everyone is different, but the voice that tries to tempt you back in, under the guise of 'Everything will be OK – you will easily be able to moderate!' seems to play upon those who are not yet 'all in' on alcohol; the jury is still out in their heads on its true effects. They are still romanticising alcohol; they are still listening to the messages that it has some upside. They are still delusional.

WHAT I LEARNT

MODERATION IS A MINDSET

There are two types of people in the moderation scenario. *The Moderation Planners* and the *Moderators*.

Firstly, the *Moderation Planners*, or aspiring moderators, have stopped drinking for a month or even longer. They believe they have cracked it and can control alcohol. They are entertaining the idea of being able to moderate and are thinking of having the odd drink, now and again.

Secondly, the *Moderators*. They claim to be able to moderate their alcohol drinking. They only drink alcohol when they want to. It's their choice. It's on their terms. They never think of alcohol outside the few times a month, or a year, that they decide they would like to have a drink or two.

The 'Mirage Of Moderation' is simply a fantasy of the *Moderation Planners* who WANT TO BELIEVE that *Moderators* do not have a problem with alcohol. They WANT TO BELIEVE that THEY will not have a problem with alcohol if they start drinking again.

What is clear about moderation is that it is not a behaviour – it's a mindset. IT'S A BELIEF. Moderation is seen as a positive ability. The ability to moderate is made up by the mind of an ex-drinker who would love to drink again but without the baggage that comes with it. A *Moderator* sounds like a fairy tale character. Maybe because it is!

We will never really know if a *Moderator* can moderate. They could all be masking the fact that they cannot live their life without alcohol.

The best way to show this is to switch what is being moderated. Let's say you met someone who told you they were moderating the number of pineapples they ate. I would immediately think, 'Why do they need to do that? Are they possibly worried that their pineapple consumption could get out of control or is it already out of control?' Let's also look at switching it to other addictive drugs like nicotine or heroin. If someone said to me they were moderating either of these, I think it would be safe to say that they either have a problem with them, or soon will!

Moderators claim they can take it or leave it; alcohol makes no difference to them. This is a stereotype and a mirage made up by the *Moderation Planner*. This is the 'Mirage of Moderation'.

DEFINING MODERATION

The dictionary says, 'Moderation is the avoidance of excess or extremes, especially in one's behaviour.' But what is excess? Excess has different levels, depending on who you are. One person may define themselves as a moderator if they drink only on Friday and/or Saturday night and special occasions. Another might define themselves as a moderator if they can go a whole year without drinking and then decide to have a few glasses of Champagne at Christmas.

WHY DO WE ENTERTAIN MODERATION?

The triggers for letting the 'Mirage of Moderation' have an impact will be different for everyone, for example: dealing with grief; dealing with a life change; dealing with fear of missing out. But the reason will always be the same: your mind has been brainwashed into thinking that alcohol will solve your problem. It will make you feel good; it will relax you; it will make you happier; it will make you a better person. This is, and always has been, a false assumption, and is a major limiting belief.

You've got to the good place of alcohol-free living and now you want to return to the place you have spent months convincing yourself is bad. If you entertain the 'Mirage of Moderation', you are just kidding yourself because the reason why you went on an alcohol-free journey was because you couldn't control alcohol consumption. You weren't very good at it then, so why do you think you'd be any good at it now, or after one year alcohol-free?

SCIENCE

To scientifically prove the case for 'moderation', we really need an independent survey of at least 50, or maybe even 100, people who have stopped drinking completely for at least a year and then decide that they will have an occasional drink. The real proof would emerge. Would they be able to moderate or would they slide back into the alcohol trap, back into the circle of addiction?

Since starting my alcohol-free journey 18 months ago, I have carried out my own research. This includes reading the posts of around 25 people who have gone over a year alcohol-free and decided to dabble again.

So far, I haven't seen anyone – online or among friends – who has been able to moderate successfully if they weren't able to do so in the first place. I do know a few people who have never drunk much and continue to drink a few times a year who I would not consider having control issues with alcohol. But I can't think of anyone who has learnt to moderate!

STEPS YOU CAN TAKE

STEP 1 – SEE IT AS A MIRAGE

Start seeing moderation for what it really is – a mirage. One of the biggest decisions I ever made was to realise this. Moderation for someone who has previously not been able to control drinking is nothing but a fantasy. Just ask the thousands who thought they could and failed!

STEP 2 – WILD CARDS DON'T WORK

Don't give yourself Wild Cards. Playing a Wild Card is a term meaning you can have a day-off. Go back to drinking for the day. No harm done. Sort of moderating.

There are a couple of people I know who gave themselves the odd Wild Card each year. What happened in both cases was that the Wild Card evolved into a 'Get Out of Jail Free Card' and instead of two or three Wild Cards a year, they were doing five or six and eventually they were back in the pit.

I've seen lots of stories recounting that as soon as people start to moderate, all the usual side effects of alcohol kick in: ruined well-being, anxiety, waking in the night, short temper and being less present.

STEP 3 – BECOME ADVERTISING AWARE

Look out for the false promises in alcohol advertising. It's hard not to when you're looking for it.

Drinking alcohol is still promoted as sexy, fun and relaxing. Watch a James Bond movie – I think he drinks around three bottles of neat Scotch in every film – and has a great life. That's the basis of the mirage. The 'Mirage of Moderation' is driven by the way society positions and accepts alcohol.

Look at smoking. It is now universally accepted that smoking is bad for you. You do not have to justify to anyone why you no longer smoke – people understand your reasons why. The days of the *Marlboro Man* and Hollywood stars smoking in every scene have gone. It is no longer fun, sexy or relaxing to smoke. There is no 'Mirage of Moderation' in the smoking world.

STEP 4 – DON'T BE DELUDED

Keep reminding yourself constantly about alcohol's false promises.

Write them down and put them where you can see them. On your fridge door. On your computer. On a Post-it note.

- Anxiety
- Sleepless nights
- Hangovers
- Anger
- Weight gain
- Huge financial cost
- Poor health

Moderation Planners are deluded. They dream of a wonderful, idyllic life where they can drink alcohol, get drunk, be happy, have fun and wake up the next day not craving it. They dream of not even thinking about it until they decide they would like it again. Their delusion is one of control. They have not fully understood the huge mountain of science that says that alcohol kills you; it's addictive; it is not fun; it does not relax you. They just have a deluded belief which they hold onto.

Anyone planning to moderate pictures themselves having a great time, laughing with friends in a pub or in a bar. They take themselves back to a time when they first started drinking alcohol, a time before it became a problem for them. They want to believe alcohol is fun. The reality is that it's a flavoured, addictive poison. Life is not like that. You can't go back to the way it was in the past. You have to find a new path, a way forward.

KEY LEARNINGS

- I haven't seen anyone who has been able to moderate successfully if they weren't able to do so in the first place.

- I can't think of anyone who has learned to moderate if they weren't able to do so in the first place!

- Is an ex-heroin addict in control of their heroin habit if they dabble once a week or maybe just on their birthday or special occasions?

- Moderation is not a behaviour. It's a mindset. It's a belief.

- Moderation is seen as a positive thing. A moderator sounds like a fairy tale character. Maybe because it is!

- 'Wild Cards' evolve into 'Get Out Of Jail Free Cards'.

- Anyone planning to moderate is deluded. They take themselves back to a time when they first started drinking alcohol, before it became a problem for them.

- Anyone planning to moderate wants to believe alcohol is fun. The reality is that it's a flavoured, addictive poison.

CHAPTER 23
THE FINAL ONE PER CENT

**To stop drinking successfully and banish
the voice that tells you that alcohol has anything good to
offer, you have to be 'All In'.**

MY STORY

It was around the seven-month mark that I slammed the door shut on any thoughts I had about not making it to 365 days, alcohol-free.

I can't pinpoint the exact date when it happened. But it happened. From that point, I had no affiliation with alcohol at all. I had completely changed my story and realised that I would live the rest of my life free of alcohol. It was one of the best feelings ever. It was so liberating.

On Day One, I had begun the process of closing the door on alcohol. My initial plan was to shut the door for 28 days. This turned into 90 days. And finally, it became forever: locking it and throwing away the key!

This final step to freedom is best explained by looking at it in percentage terms:

On Day One, I slammed the door completely shut with the intention of making it to my first target of 28 days sober. By Day Four, however, it had started to open. The first three days' honeymoon was over and the door was now slightly ajar; let's say 5% open. This was only natural. I had been drinking almost every day for 35 years, so doubt was naturally going to creep into my head. Over the first few weeks, the voices were tempting me to have a drink. When they did, the door swung further ajar, to around 10 to 15% open.

By Month Seven, the door was 99% closed. But there was still the odd doubt in my mind, questioning whether I could get to 365 days and beyond, plus the occasional craving once or twice a week.

I needed to lock the door. I did this by revisiting my 'Whys' – the reasons why I was here in the first place. It's easy to get flippant about them but do so at the risk of upsetting the whole process.

WHAT I LEARNT

SHUT THAT DOOR

As long as doubt is there, there is still a slim chance that you could be pushed, jump or even fall 'off the wagon'.

To close and lock the door you have to go 'All In'. This is a poker term for putting all your money on your hand because you firmly believe you will win the game. 'All In' is what it says – it is not 50%, 70% and 99%. It's 100%. You are prepared to give all your energy to achieving the goal.

If you really think about it, there is no difference between being 50% committed and 99% committed. In both scenarios, you are not fully committed and still open to possible failure.

When you're 'All In', you are fully committed. When this happens, everything becomes easy. I believe that I had read so much Quit Lit, and gone so many days along the alcohol-free road, that I started to truly believe that my life is better without alcohol.

I had trodden a new pathway in my mind that had become permanent. I no longer needed any willpower because there was no longer anything to give up. It was history.

All the skills I was learning, including understanding habit loops, dealing with cravings, building my new values, questioning my beliefs and purpose, were slowly, but surely, pushing the door back to closed. Seven months in, I found the final 1%, locked the door and threw away the key.

This last one per cent was the most challenging. It represented the doubt that existed somewhere deep in my mind that I might fail.

It is so important to understand this and get rid of this doubt, because if not killed off, it could grow. This is what I believe happens to people who go back to moderating. They leave the door unlocked and keep hold of the key to unlock it.

STEPS YOU CAN TAKE

STEP 1 – GET WISE ABOUT YOUR 'WHYS'

To go 'All In' and achieve the final 1%, review why you started this journey in the first place. Get wise about your 'Whys'. Look at your original 'Whys'. These will be the reasons that get you over the finish line.

KEY LEARNINGS

- This 'final one per cent' is challenging. It represents the doubt that exists somewhere deep in your mind that you might fail.

- To go 'All In' and achieve the final one per cent, review why you started this journey in the first place. Look at your original 'Whys'.

CHAPTER 24
COMING OUT

When you stop drinking, several obstacles come up time and time again:

- *How to tell the world you no longer drink*
- *How to deal with social gatherings where you would normally drink*
- *What to say to others who ask why you're not drinking*

MY STORY

For the first three months, I didn't tell anyone outside my close family that I had stopped drinking. It was only from around 90 days onwards that I started telling a few close friends and work colleagues.

The reasons were a mixture of the embarrassment and fear of failure that are built into many people's journeys.

In the last few years of drinking, I felt shame and embarrassment that I'd let alcohol get control. It was this shame that stayed with me well into my alcohol-free journey. By telling the outside world that I had stopped drinking, I believed I was admitting that I had a problem of control. Well, that's what I thought.

There was also the fear of failure – the fear of 'losing face' if I was not able to reach the 28-day, 90-day, and 365-day alcohol-free targets. I thought it would be better not to tell anybody than tell the world and possibly fail!

In the past, I found it hard to stop drinking for these reasons, so I just carried on because it's easier just to keep on doing what you're doing: 'Better the devil you know!'

As I got more days under my belt and became more confident in my abilities to break my habit, I started to tell a few more people each week.

Around the six-month mark, my journey had become firmly centred around my health and fitness, driven by my 9KM BY 9AM adventure. I was walking 9km every day before 9am, so I created social media pages dedicated to this and my wider journey.

It was through these pages that I started to openly tell the world about the fact that I was a non-drinker. The pages and posts are a fly-on-the-wall documentary of my journey, where I talk about my alcohol-free life and give tips and insights for others who are considering stopping drinking.

I guess it was a lot easier to 'come out of the alcohol closet' as 9KM BY 9AM, not Nigel Jones.

I felt that once I had achieved 365 days, both embarrassment and fear would have been resolved. No embarrassment because I obviously now had control. No fear of failure because I had not failed. I also believed that one year alcohol-free sounded a thousand times more credible than six or seven months.

With hindsight, this is all complete rubbish that my ego was making up. It was the story in my head that I had created. I had known at around seven months in that I had beaten the booze. The fact that I had kept the story back from the rest of my world because of embarrassment and fear was crazy.

On my personal social media pages, I kept things quiet until just a few days before I reached 365 days. I was planning on an announcement to everyone on the 365th day but I just could not wait and let it slip out in a video on my personal Facebook page around 10 days before the big day.

The response was fantastic. So many people said, 'Well done!', that they were proud of me and that I inspired them. It really meant the world to me. It was this response that made me realise that I enjoyed helping others and that I should pursue a career in life coaching, helping people with alcohol control.

My approach felt right for me even though I can now see it does not matter what other people think. Do it for yourself and your loved ones.

DEALING WITH SOCIAL GATHERINGS

In terms of social gatherings and events, this was not a problem for me because I stopped drinking in the middle of the pandemic. So, for most of my first year alcohol-free, there weren't many social gatherings and events because of lockdowns and social distancing.

Of the few I attended, I always planned ahead. Here's what I did:

- I called the pub or restaurant ahead of the event and asked what AF options they had, so it wasn't a surprise when I arrived and found out they didn't have any!

- For house parties and get-togethers, I took my own AF drinks. Otherwise, I would have been drinking cola all night!

- If the event was solely based around drinking, for example, a pub crawl – I didn't go.

WHAT TO SAY

I never went out of my way to announce I was a non-drinker or force my opinions on others about all the facts I had discovered.

I think that's the worst thing you can do as it draws attention to yourself and can wind people up, particularly if they have a drink in their hand and are out 'enjoying' themselves. No-one wants to know that the drink they have is poison and kills millions of people every year!

I simply said I'd stopped drinking for health reasons and I was feeling so much better as a result.

This often prompted the response, from a few people, that they 'did not drink much' and so 'did not need to stop' because their health was OK!

I also found that stopping drinking is like holding a mirror up to others. They would immediately reflect on their own drinking habits and try and put me into a box that makes them feel comfortable. For example: 'Did you have a problem?' (No, I didn't have a problem); 'Did you do it for health reasons?' (No, I am healthy); 'Have you gone crazy?' (No, I am not mad).

If anyone was inquisitive and wanted to find out more, I'd let them know my story, mindful of the fact that if they had a drink in their hand, it was a better move to keep it 'topline' or change the subject.

Now in my second year alcohol-free, I just say 'I don't drink alcohol', without an explanation.

People who did not know me when I was drinking, normally don't ask further, as they only know me as a non-drinker, and it could sound rude to start probing. This also works for those I have known longer. I say, 'I stopped drinking alcohol.'

WHAT I LEARNT

A few things that stand out are:

There is no reason to be embarrassed or fearful. You are the trailblazer. You are the one that has opened your eyes and seen that you have been lied to about alcohol all your life. There is nothing wrong with stopping killing yourself. There is nothing wrong in wanting to escape the lies that most people have succumbed to and continue to put up with day in, day out.

As time goes by, and you become totally alcohol-free, everybody will know you are a non-drinker and the challenges presented early on subside, then go away.

When people make the fact that you aren't drinking 'a thing', it's simply because something within them, consciously or subconsciously, is calling them to examine their own relationship with alcohol.

Don't overthink it. You don't need to explain yourself for not drinking any more than the person asking does for drinking.

STEPS YOU CAN TAKE

STEP 1 – KNOW THE REASONS WHY YOU'RE NOT DRINKING

If anyone asks you why you're not drinking, you could use any one of the following, from the table below, depending on how deeply you want to go into the explanation. I have also set out some typical responses I got.

Your response should be dependent on the situation. If the other person is drinking, my advice is to hold back. You could get into an inflamed dialogue, simply because you could find yourself up against their limiting belief that 'alcohol is good for you'.

ANSWERS	TYPICAL RESPONSE
KEEP IT SIMPLE I don't drink.	Most people won't ask the reason. If they do, you just say, 'It doesn't agree with me.'
DON'T LIKE IT I don't like alcohol.	This tends to move the conversation on.

GENERAL HEALTH It just wasn't doing my health any good.	Most people will ask 'Do you feel better?' Some start talking about their own drinking and asking your opinion. Typically: 'I've been thinking of cutting it out. Was it hard?' (No) 'Do you feel like you are missing out?' (No, I have yet to feel like I am missing out.) 'Do you just drink boring soft drinks?' (No, there are loads of AF drinks now.)
SPECIFIC HEALTH I stopped because… choose one or more of the following: - It causes cancer, liver disease, etc. - It makes me fat. - I hate hangovers. - I want to live longer. - It makes me drowsy. - It fuels my anxiety.	This tends to move the conversation on – quicker for more serious ailments!
CHALLENGE I'm on a health challenge, which you are. - I'm doing a 28-day challenge. - I'm following a self-care programme and it includes no alcohol. - I like to get up early to see the sunrise each morning.	This will turn the conversation to your challenge and not drinking.
MONETARY I am saving the money I would have spent on alcohol towards a family holiday later in the year.	This could take you into a whole conversation about how much money you spend and they spend on alcohol.
DRIVING I'm driving or I'm the designated driver.	This tends to move the conversation on.

MORE IN-DEPTH ANSWERS If you feel you want to say something about not drinking, keep it simple: - It gives me headaches, interferes with my sleep, etc. - It wakes me up during the night with dry mouth and headache.	This could lead to a full-on discussion. If that is what you want, then going into depth in your answer will achieve this. Share your story if you feel like doing so but if you don't, simply state: I don't drink; it doesn't agree with me.
SMUG ANSWER Say, been there, got the t-shirt. Just decided to stop and I feel amazing!	Not advisable to people you do not know or have an alcoholic beverage in their hand! This is red rag to a bull territory.
WHITE LIE Sometimes you may feel it is appropriate to make up a reason, such as, I'm taking antibiotics.	Most people don't question this and feel sorry for you because you can't drink!

STEP 2 – GOING TO A PARTY TIPS

In the early days, it's important to have a plan in place that covers: which gatherings you want to go to; what you're going to drink there; what you're going to say if you are asked why you don't drink.

Here are some Dos and Don'ts for parties, social gatherings and occasions where there could be alcohol present:

DO

• Visualise the experience.

• Be proud that you are alcohol-free.

• Take some alcohol-free drinks with you.

• Be honest – always the best way forward and you'll feel much better and relieved for it!

• Be present, in the moment, enjoy it. If you're not having fun, make your excuses and leave.

DON'T

- Be a bull in a china shop, showing off about your alcohol-free status. Remember, a couple of drinks in and no-one notices who's drinking and who isn't.

KEY LEARNINGS

- For some, it's hard to stop drinking because of shame, embarrassment and fear of failure. They just carry on because it's easier just to keep on doing what they're doing.

- For others, telling the outside world that they have stopped drinking is effectively admitting that they have a problem of control.

- Stopping drinking can be like holding a mirror up. Many people immediately reflect on their own drinking habits and try and put you into a box that makes them feel comfortable.

- When people make the fact that you aren't drinking 'a thing', it's simply because something within them is calling them to examine their own relationship with alcohol.

- Don't overthink the answer you give to, 'Why are you not drinking?'

- You don't need to explain yourself for not drinking any more than the person asking needs to explain why they are drinking.

CHAPTER 25
IF YOU FALL 'OFF THE WAGON'

'It's not what happens to you, but how you react that matters.' **Epictetus**

MY STORY

'On the wagon' is a phrase used to describe someone who is abstaining from drinking any alcoholic drink, usually in the sense of having given it up, as opposed to never having drunk alcohol. 'Off the wagon' describes someone who is no longer abstaining.

Over 35 years of drinking, the longest I stayed on the wagon was six days. I tried hundreds of times to jump back on but always fell off again.

This time around, I have never once left the wagon and have absolutely no plans ever to do so again. At the time of writing this, I stopped drinking over 500 days ago and alcohol is now firmly something I did in a past life.

My advice on what to do if you fall off the wagon is based on what I observed, reading the stories of hundreds of people who started out with long-term intentions of alcohol-free living. Some managed to get back on, but others fell by the wayside.

There is definitely a correlation between wanting to go back to drinking alcohol and the length of time spent away from it. I was tempted in the early days, but the longer I went into the journey, the further I travelled away from my old drinking lifestyle and the easier it became to stay alcohol-free.

Once I had got past seven days, 14 days became the target, then 28, then 90, then 200, then 365.

For the majority that managed to make it past 90 days, it was a lot easier to get back on the wagon than for those with less alcohol-free days under their belts.

That's not the full story, however. My observations of how easy or difficult it is to get back on the wagon are dependent not just on how long you have been on it, but also on your understanding of how you left the wagon in the first place!

WAYS TO FALL OFF THE WAGON

At first glance, it seems there are several ways I could leave the wagon. I could jump off, fall off, get pulled off or be pushed off!

If I decided to jump, it's my choice. Yes, I might well be influenced by others, but it would be me who would take this final decision.

If I fell off, it would be my choice again because I can only fall off if I'm too close to the edge, or too close to wanting to drink. I would have been careless to put myself in this position. There's a great saying, 'If you hang around the barber's shop long enough, you're going to get a haircut.'

If I was pulled off, it would be because I would have given in to friends who are off the wagon; who beckoned me to come and join them. Or I would have allowed societal pressure, which continually tells me that being off the wagon is a good thing, to get to me.

If I got pushed off, I would have been influenced by someone on the wagon with me. This can happen when a couple both stop drinking and one of them decides to have a drink, thereby pushing or influencing the other to come along for the ride and give it a go. I am lucky that this never happened to me because my wife does not drink!

But on further inspection, I soon realised that there is only one way that I would leave the wagon and that is through my own choice. It is no one else's fault. I am the master of my own destiny. No-one can make me drink alcohol unless they put a gun to my head.

This point is crucial to making it a much easier process to getting back on the wagon. You have to realise that it's your own doing. You are the only one responsible. Once you understand this, the method I prescribe below to get back on – and stay on – will work.

WHAT I LEARNT

THE WAGON IS MOVING

Moderation is the belief you can jump on the wagon and off the wagon whenever and wherever you want, and still be in complete control of your relationship with alcohol.

If the wagon is stationary, jumping on and off would not be hard. But can you imagine how difficult it would be if the wagon is moving, and not just moving slowly, but at speed. It would require a superpower to be able to do this.

My assumption that the wagon moves is founded on the fact that a wagon has wheels – otherwise the saying would be I'm 'on the static cart', which doesn't have the same ring to it.

If you were able to get back on, you would more than likely hurt yourself in the process. Or even worse, you would end up falling and watching it disappear into the distance, as you drop back into your life off the wagon, and potentially into a cycle of alcohol addiction. You may not even get the chance to try and jump back on because the wagon has already left and is nowhere in sight!

DON'T JUST BE ON THE WAGON!

I like to think of myself as not just being on the wagon but upfront driving it, or even in a room inside the wagon with a locked door. I don't intend to get off it at all. I think that's important because once you've made that decision to stay on the wagon, life is better and fuller; you have escaped the hamster wheel of continually jumping on and off the wagon.

STEPS YOU CAN TAKE

If you jump off the wagon and realise it was a big mistake to do so, you need to jump back on immediately.

If you are planning to jump off, or have already jumped off, my suggestion is to do the following:

STEP 1 – GET BACK ON

The first thing you need to do is get back on. Call it what you want. A new Day One or a continuation of where you got to before you left. It does not matter. All that matters is that you get back to being alcohol-free.

STEP 2 – FOLLOW THE METHOD

The method needed to make your transition back to being on the wagon as quick and easy as possible is the same method you took to get on it in the first place. That's how you get back safely on the wagon.

In no order:

Revisit Your Whys – go back to why you decided to be alcohol-free. For me it is to:

- be healthier – to minimise risk of cancer, liver problems, heart disease, etc.
- lose and maintain a healthy weight; to look better and be able to wear nicer clothes.
- not look like I am a drinker!

- have a better and more fulfilling relationship with my family – my wife, my children and my mother.

Re-read your Quit Lit – reinforce your new beliefs about alcohol. You had a slip-up, but that's all it was. All the truths you learnt about alcohol are still the same – less anxiety, better sleep, more money, better relationships... the list is endless.

Revisit your Values, Beliefs and Purpose – values motivate your actions and help you make decisions. The person I want to be for the rest of my life is a healthy, fit, calm, caring, successful, hardworking, family-orientated, happily-married person. Being alcohol-free is central to my beliefs and purpose. So, I would simply ask myself, 'Would someone with these values want to go back to drinking alcohol?' The answer is no.

Revisit The Habit Loop – look again at the habit loop. There are three parts to the habit loop: the cue or trigger that kicks off the habitual behaviour; the routine or the habit or repeated behaviour; and the reward. Identify the reason why your craving was triggered and ensure it does not happen again.

Understand your Cravings – remember that cravings are like waves. Each has a start. Some are bigger than others. Some last longer than others. What they all have in common is they all end when they crash on the shore.

Remember Moderation is a Mirage – I haven't seen anyone who has been able to moderate successfully if they weren't able to do so in the first place. Anyone planning to moderate is deluded. They want to believe alcohol is fun. The reality is it's a flavoured, addictive poison.

Practise The Mindfulness of Intention – become aware of intention before you act. This will enable you to make wise choices that lead you to clarity, well-being, and harmony. Without awareness of intention, you can easily end up reacting, living on autopilot or mindlessly following old habits. Observing your mind closely, you'll see that intention precedes every action.

'*Premeditatio Malorum*' – the premeditation of evils. This Stoic saying means appreciate and be grateful for what you have. Imagine that everything that can go wrong will go wrong. Make plans so you know what to do to stop yourself jumping off.

STEP 3 – SLAM THE DOOR SHUT

The fact that you jumped off the wagon or are planning to jump off is because you are close to the edge. This represents the fact that you still somewhere, deep in your mind, believe alcohol has an upside.

Imagine a room on the wagon. By following Step 2, you will be able to enter the room and firmly shut and lock the door behind you and throw away the key.

KEY LEARNINGS

- There is a correlation between wanting to go back to drinking alcohol and time spent away from it.

- For the majority that manage to make it past 90 days, it is a lot easier to get back on the wagon than for those with less alcohol-free days under their belts.

- There's really only one way to leave the wagon and that's through your own choice. It's no one else's fault. You are the master of your own destiny. No-one can make you drink alcohol.

- If you are planning to jump off, or have already jumped off, the first thing you need to do is get back on. Call it what you want. A new Day One or a continuation of where you got to before you left. It does not matter. All that matters is that you get back to being alcohol-free.

- The method needed to make your transition back to being on the wagon as quick and easy as possible is the same method you took to get on it in the first place. That's how you get safely back on the wagon.

- The fact that you jumped off the wagon, or are planning to jump off, is because you got close to the edge. This represents the fact that you still somewhere, deep in your mind, believe alcohol has an upside.

- Imagine a room on the wagon. Enter the room and firmly shut and lock the door behind you and throw away the key.

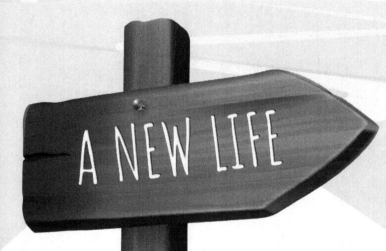

A NEW LIFE

ONE YEAR
& BEYOND

A NEW LIFE:
ONE YEAR & BEYOND

If you don't have a plan, someone will have a plan for you.

Imagine asking the captain of a ship, 'Where are you heading?' and they say, 'I don't know.'

This is the same as having no goals to aim for, no targets. You end up rudderless in a sea of other people's dreams and ambitions.

This section shows what it's like on the other side of 365 Days alcohol-free.

It explores how I felt about myself a year in, what others thought of me, and my plans and dreams for the rest of my life.

CHAPTER 26
MY NEW LIFE

Mark Twain famously said, 'The two most important days of your life are the day you are born and the day you find out why.'

MY STORY

I woke up on Day 366 a different person. I could see clearly now the booze had gone.

A superpower had unleashed within me. A clarity had built up over the whole year, but on Day One of Year Two, it was firmly part of my belief system.

Even though I had closed the door on alcohol at around 200 days in, on Day 366, I had not only closed that door, but I had also locked it and thrown away the key.

The anxiety, hangovers and not remembering what I said or did the night before, had gone. There was a new clarity to my life. The sleepless nights, sweats, and the endless list of the negative effects of alcohol on my well-being, were no longer my problem.

I could see my authentic self. All the crap of pretending to be somebody I wasn't, had gone for good.

Today, I know my values, my beliefs, and my purpose. I have changed, both mentally and physically. This was not overnight; it was a process that had taken a whole year.

It is so worth it. I would not swap my first year alcohol-free for anything. I would go back and live it again if I could. It was not an easy time; it was not a tough time, but it was above everything else the best year of my life simply because I found out who I am. And I did this by stopping drinking.

On Day One, a major part of my 'new' values was the fact that I'd stopped drinking. This was now a major part of who I was. 'I've stopped drinking. I used to drink but I don't drink any more.' This was part of my new identity – it defined me. Every day I was telling myself, 'I have stopped drinking. I'm no longer a drinker and I am on a journey to alcohol freedom.'

I was, effectively, a work in progress. I was not yet a 100% non-drinker. What was still defining me was the fact that I had stopped. I was in between being a drinker and a fully-fledged non-drinker.

The longer I went into the journey, the greater the fear became of going back to where I had come from. I felt I had more to lose, simply because of all the effort that I had put into stopping drinking alcohol. If I succumbed, all the days that I had accumulated would have been a waste of time!

But there came a point when I woke up and saw clearly for the first time. This is a wonderful experience. The best experience ever. This started to happen for me after around 200 days but by Day 365, I really could see clearly now the booze had gone.

The fact that I don't drink has become a part of me. I have none of the fear of going back to drinking. It's not something I'm actively doing and it's not something I think about any more. I just don't drink. It's no longer on my agenda.

It truly is a wonderful place to be. It's the place that I wanted to be when I set out on the journey. Now I am here; it is true enlightenment.

WHAT'S CHANGED?

There are so many changes for the good that stand out, but here's my Top 10! These are the reasons I feel so empowered post-365 days.

AUTHENTIC-SELF & PURPOSE – Being alcohol-free has allowed me to understand my values, my beliefs, and my purpose. Using these three measures, I created a mindset, a vision, a mission, that led me to a fulfilling life filled with fun and happiness. My mind is not clouded any more. I've walked away from the limiting beliefs that were holding me back. One of the major changes I made was to my belief system, making THERE IS NOTHING I CAN'T DO a central part of who I am. Setting goals and following my dreams became a lot easier when I knew my values, beliefs, and purpose. I'm still getting to know myself and I much prefer the new authentic, real me. He was always there; I just did not know how to find him.

CONTROL – I am in control. I am the master of my destiny. Old me had become way too much influenced by alcohol. It had crept into almost everything I did. It was like an invisible hand, helping me make decisions. I deluded myself for years that I was in control, creating scenarios like:

Let's go to that hotel (reason – because the bar is great). Let's go on that walk (reason – because there's a pub I like along the way). Let's leave at that time (reason – as the pub will be open by the time we get there). At its core, alcohol-free living means that I am the sole decision-maker. It is me who decides how I spend my one 'wild and precious life'. I can drive anywhere I want, on any night of the week.

SELF RESPECT – I respect myself more now I am alcohol-free. I am more aware of myself because I am more present and I'm not taking my mind to some other place. I am very rarely tired. I am full of energy and have a 'get up and go' attitude to almost everything. All these things led me to put more focus on myself, my diet, my skin, my fitness, and my general well-being.

RESPECT FOR OTHERS – Through respecting myself, I soon started to respect others more. This is like a positive gratitude feedback loop. The more I gave, the better I felt, so the more I gave. I absolutely love it if I find out my journey has inspired other people. This is a core part of my purpose.

CLARITY – I thought I knew who and what was important to me. It was not until I stopped drinking that I realised how flawed this view was. Alcohol is an imposter that causes fear and anxiety. It took me away from the present moment and the real world. Being alcohol-free definitely gives me more clarity. I live more in the now, and the now is where things happen. They don't happen in the past!

RESPOND NOT REACT – By learning how to be more present in my mind, I am now less likely to get caught up in stories in my head or fall into reactive patterns of behaviour like arguing and making poor choices. Mindfulness practice taught me how to build a 'window of reaction', the time between something happening that could affect me and my response to it. There are thousands of examples, but let's take one where a lot of us might normally 'lose it':

While driving my car, someone overtakes me and cuts in front of me. One reaction might be to go into full-on road rage. Another, and the New Me way, would just simply put it down to the fact that the other driver must have something pressing on his mind, and I wish him a great day.

If you can control the reaction to a stimulus, you are pretty much in control of your destiny. Seriously.

AF MEANS ANXIETY FREE – Anxiety for me is pretty much a thing of the past. Alcohol took me away from the present and to the world of fretting about the future or worrying over things that had already happened. I trained myself to clear my mind of past or future thoughts and just think of what is now. To get back to the present, I use mindfulness and compassion to address my fears. I love Yoda's quote, 'Named must your fear be, before banish it you can.'

HEALTH – I haven't felt as fit as I do today since my 20s. After nine months of being alcohol-free, I was called in for my five-year NHS Health Check. The results showed that I had lost three stone in weight; my blood pressure was 115/80; my cholesterol was 3.49; and my overall risk of cardiovascular disease in the next 10 years was 5.1%. I was aware from Day One that I had to up my game physically and exercise more. I also knew I had to take a serious look at my diet. This was all driven by the fact that I had stopped drinking. Well-being doors were opening up every day for me. I just wanted to be healthier; it was becoming a self-fulfilling prophecy. The real magic, in the form of significant weight loss, started to happen from six months onwards, after I started the 9KM BY 9AM walks.

FITNESS – I would now consider myself fit. It sounds weird to me saying that. But it is true. I started walking daily at the beginning of the journey and six months in created 9KM BY 9AM. Each day, I walk at least 9km before 9am – whatever the weather! After 11 months, I have walked over 330 days, covering on average over 10km per day, totalling around 3,000kms. This is the equivalent of around 75 marathons – and all before breakfast! For me, 9KM BY 9AM is a metaphor. It's about doing something challenging early in the day.

SLEEP – I need six and a half to seven hours per night. I'm wide awake after that. For the past nine months or so, I've been fast asleep between 10.15pm and 4.45am. The early morning feeling is one of the best feelings I have ever had: the feeling of being ready for the day, excited to get out of bed. Now, well into Year Two of no alcohol, it is still my favourite time of the day. It's a time when I can get things done.

Most of all, I am proud of myself that I don't drink. I am proud to be part of a growing community of like-minded people who have chosen to live life without alcohol.

IMPACT ON OTHERS

A huge eye-opener was not just how I thought I had changed, but what others close to me thought of the new me. I am not talking about the physical changes, which are clear to see, but about how I changed inside.

My friends say I am more myself, more confident and more authentic; more caring about both myself, my personal health and them. They also noticed that I have become more go-getting. If I want to do something, I just do it.

My wife and children are all very proud of me, scoring me 10 out of 10 on the proud scale. My wife says I am thinner and have nicer skin but am still ugly! The major change she has seen is that I am more in touch with reality, more present and appreciate nature and what is around me more. She says that I have embraced the alcohol-free and vegetarian ways of life; I eat better; I see the benefits of eating more fruit and vegetables. I also don't smell of alcohol and I remember what she tells me!

My three children, who are in their late teens and early twenties, scored me 8.5 out of 10 for calmness; 8 out of 10 for caring; and 8 out of 10 for loving. A few quotes from them are:

- 'I am very proud of you. All my friends are very impressed when I tell them what you have achieved and what you do every day.'
- 'You're happier, and I argue less with you.'
- 'You appreciate life more and are passionate about what you do.'
- 'You're more tolerable.'

I will take this last one as a real positive!

My 90-year-old mother says, 'I admire you for what you have made of your life. I find you very kind and very caring. What else can I ask for?'

WHAT I LEARNT

THE POWER OF DÉJÀ VU

The thing about Day 366 is that it feels like you're used to it. The same is true for every day in Year Two. Been there; done that.

After 365 days, each new day is a day that you've done before, each month is a month you've done before. This had a very powerful effect on me. It gave me confidence. January is not a problem because I was alcohol-free last January. March is not a problem because I was alcohol-free last March. It feels like I know what I'm doing and I'm completely 100% in control.

COUP D'ÉTAT

By Day 366, I had put in place a new government to run my mind and body for the rest of my days on this planet. But, as with all good plans, I knew that for this coup to be successful and the new government to stay in power, I needed to ensure I had the firepower to win and a solid base for this new government to grow on.

Put simply, I was going to need a new set of ministers to run a whole new set of departments. Being alcohol-free meant I had more energy, was more aware of my mind and body, was more present and less anxious. I also slept better and wanted to learn more. Stopping drinking had freed up so much time, which would have been lost to watching TV, talking nonsense in bars, getting up late with a headache and spending far too much time stressing over the past or worrying about the future.

So, the new main departments were: Physical Health & Fitness; Mental Well-being; Nutrition; Sleep; Education. With my enlightened ego running each of these departments, and the New Me as both the Prime Minister and Head of State, it could not fail.

STEPS YOU CAN TAKE

STEP 1 – IF YOU ARE JUST STARTING OUT OR ARE MAKING YOUR WAY DOWN THE ROAD

If you have jumped to the end of the book and have either not yet started your journey or are somewhere along the road, my suggestion is:

- Read this book. Split into six parts, it follows my experiences over the first year of alcohol-free living. Each chapter has a STEPS YOU CAN TAKE section at the end, to help you on your journey. Hopefully, there will be a few nuggets in there that will help you reach Day 366.

- Start now – today! – if you are still contemplating. *Memento Mori.*

- Take a Challenge and evolve it: 7 days, 28 days, 90 days, 365 days.

- Join the AF community – there are hundreds of groups. Start talking to others also following an AF lifestyle.

STEP 2 – IF YOU HAVE COMPLETED A YEAR

If you are reading this and you have completed 365 days, many, many congratulations! My suggestion is:

- Keep going. I never felt the need to moderate. The benefits of being alcohol-free are just too huge. Even one drink is simply not worth it.

- Enjoy your one wonderful life!

KEY LEARNINGS

- I woke up on Day 366 and was a different person.
- I could see my authentic self. All the crap of pretending to be somebody I wasn't had gone for good.

- There came a point when I woke up and saw clearly for the first time that I am alcohol-free. This started to happen for me at around 200 days.

- The fact that I don't drink has become a part of me. It's not something I'm actively doing and it's not something I think about any more. I just don't drink. It's no longer on my agenda.

- Alcohol-free is truly a wonderful place to be. It's the place that I wanted to be when I set out on the journey. Now I am here, it is true enlightenment.

- The thing about Day 366 is that it feels like you're used to it. The same is true for every day in Year Two. Been there; done that.

- I am proud of myself that I don't drink. I am proud that I am part of a growing community of like-minded people who have chosen to live life without alcohol.

CHAPTER 27
POST 365 – WHAT'S NEXT?

Imagine if the astronauts who went to the moon did not tell anybody anything about what they learnt there – not one iota!

MY STORY

My journey began in a world where I was not in control of alcohol. I left that world to learn how to follow an alcohol-free life, where my old beliefs became a thing of the past, and the familiar rules that I used to live my life by, faded away.

In this new world, I faced many obstacles and tests. Through identifying the values and beliefs I wanted to live by, I forged my new purpose and eventually earned the reward – the superpower of alcohol freedom.

But what next? What can I do with this superpower and all this knowledge? The answer is very simple. I want to share it with as many people as possible and by doing so, help others find and release their superpower.

THE WORLD'S MY OYSTER

My plan for 366 days onwards, is to follow my purpose statement, namely, that I am a healthy, sober, family man who loves learning about life, arts, culture and helping people find well-being.

Three major beliefs pretty much drive me and support my purpose.

Two of these beliefs I have had since childhood, and they still play a major part of who I am today:

'The world is my oyster!' and,

'Luck is where hard work and opportunity meet!'

Both of these remind me so much of alcohol freedom.

My mother said to me many times, 'The world is your oyster', so it stuck as a belief. I took it as meaning that everything is open to me if I persist. All oysters can be opened if I try hard enough and, if I am lucky, I could find a pearl.

But to really understand me, you have to understand what I mean by luck. I have always thought of myself as a lucky person who has done well out of life. I have always worked hard at everything I do, from school exams to part-time jobs, from running my own companies, to hobbies and interests. Things weren't just given to me. They happened because I worked hard at them and in doing so, my path crossed the paths of others who provided me with the openings or opportunities to succeed. This is what I define as luck.

The third major belief, which I added since going alcohol-free, is:

'Anything is possible'.

By passing the internal winning post of 365 days alcohol-free, I proved to myself that if I wanted it, and believed that I could do it, then I could achieve anything. Put simply – anything is possible, by believing anything is possible.

This alcohol-free journey has taken me to a place I have never been to before and I love everything about it. It has led me to a pearl, the superpower of alcohol-freedom. But I know there are more out there just waiting to be found and I am going to keep looking for them until the day I die.

My plan for the future is:

SPREADING THE ALCOHOL-FREE WORD

The central part of my purpose is to give back. I know I am not the first, and I will certainly not be the last, to learn the secret of alcohol-free living and write about it. At my core, I believe I have a duty to pass on this information as I have tried my best to do in the pages of this book.

LIFE COACHING

As well as sharing the secret in this book, I plan to help others through coaching and mentoring. I have just completed an International Coaching Federation-accredited Diploma in Positive Psychology Coaching. I plan to help anyone interested in taking a break from alcohol to hone their values, beliefs and goals, to find their purpose and to aid their well-being, self-development and positive change.

One style of coaching I use says that everyone views the world in a unique way, based on their values and beliefs. This is their unique map of life, and no two maps are the same.

Your map is not the territory. It is just the way you view the world. So, for example, someone with a map that is made up of beliefs including, '*alcohol is fun and makes you happy*', might look at a glass of wine as something that will take all their problems away. Another person's map comprising beliefs including, '*alcohol is poison and will kill you if not controlled*', will look at the same glass of wine in a very different way.

Life is full of opportunities and my plan is to help people unravel their maps, and find the treasures they seek, and understand that their futures have not yet been written.

9KM BY 9AM

Being alcohol-free means that I naturally have more energy and want to live a healthy, long life. So, I will continue with the 9KM BY 9AM scaffolding I have put around myself. I may not carry on walking 9km before 9am EVERY DAY, but I know I will be exercising daily and be involved in some form of challenge that is good for my well-being.

FUTURE BOOKS

Most of this book was written on the 9KM BY 9AM walks. I love the early mornings and the opportunity offered by those first hours of the day. I am currently writing my second book, details of which will be announced soon.

STAYING HAPPY

This book is about how I found happiness. This quest was kickstarted by taking alcohol out of my life. The one thing I gave everything up for, was now the one thing I gave up to get everything back.

What's next is all about staying happy. I will do this by following my purpose and not making the mistakes I made before. Central to my plan is staying sober. This works for me, so why break it? I know it is impossible to predict 100% that I will never drink again. I just take one day at a time. If you wake up each day and you don't want to drink, then this will mean you never drink again.

WHAT I LEARNT

If I had to pick the main things I learnt on this journey, they would be:

DO IT NOW, DO IT RIGHT NOW

It really does not matter how old you are. The best time to stop drinking is now. Arthur C. Brooks wrote that if you look at your adult life as spanning 70 years – from ages of 20 to 90 – at 45 years old, you have around 65% of your adult life left. At 55, you have 50%, and at 65 you have 35%. This is a great way of looking at it. Basically, it's never too late. Live life positively.

HELP OTHERS DISCOVER THEMSELVES

On this journey of discovery, look at yourself as a work in progress. The path will lead you to many huge achievements, which you would have settled for when you started out. But you have to keep moving on. The future will be full of adventures where you are chasing the next dream. That's the fun of all this – there is always another challenge. That's the beauty of life.

In his Oscar-winning acceptance speech in 2014, Matthew McConaughey said he has three things that he needs each day: something to look up to; another to look forward to; and another to chase. He says it is his hero that he chases. At age 15, he told his friend, who had asked him who his hero was, that his hero is himself in ten years' time. When he turned 25, that same person asked him if he is the hero. McConaughey said, 'Not even close! My hero is me at 35. You see, every day, and every week, and every month, and every year of my life, my hero is always ten years away. I'm never going to be my hero. I'm not going to obtain that... and that's fine with me because it keeps me with somebody to keep on chasing.'

NO REGRETS

Don't regret anything. Don't become an 'I coulda, I shoulda, I woulda' person. Bronnie Ware is an Australian nurse who spent many years working in palliative care, looking after patients in the last 12 weeks of their lives. In her book, *The Top Five Regrets of the Dying*, she says these regrets included:

- *Wishing I had the courage to live a life true to myself, not the life others expected of me.*
- *Wishing I'd had the courage to express my feelings.*
- *Wishing I had stayed in touch with my friends.*
- *Wishing I had let myself be happier.*
- *Wishing I hadn't worked so hard.*

You have the time now to ensure you minimise any of these potential regrets.

WHAT IS HAPPINESS?

This book is about how I became happy again, a feeling I had not had on an on-going basis since I was a child or – put another way – before I started drinking.

I truly believe that alcohol not only takes away happiness but prevents people from being happy.

But what is happiness? Martin Seligman, the father of Positive Psychology, says happiness, or as he calls it, well-being, is akin to flourishing. He developed the PERMA theory to define it.

There are five building blocks that enable flourishing: Positive Emotion, Engagement, Relationships, Meaning and Accomplishment. And there are techniques to increase each. Different people will derive happiness or well-being from each of these five blocks to varying degrees.

A good life for one person is not necessarily a good life for another. There are many different routes to a flourishing life. Here is a brief definition of each of the five building blocks:

- **Positive Emotion.** The moments when you laugh and feel joy are beautiful but are just one element of happiness or well-being. Happiness is not all about the positive emotions of laughter or buying something new. Many of us are chasing the wrong things in search of happiness. New clothes, houses, cars, material items produce momentary bursts of happiness only.

- **Engagement.** This is when you are totally absorbed in what you are doing. You are 'in the zone'. You are fully engaged in the activity with your mind and body. Sport, ballet, painting, studying and lots of our hobbies can produce these feelings. Wherever you find engagement, you can find more happiness.

- **Relationships**. Cultivating positive relationships with friends and family leads to more happiness.

- **Meaning**. This is like the engine driving happiness. Believing in a cause, or something bigger than oneself, can produce deep meaning and happiness.

- **Accomplishment**. We are designed to accomplish things even for their own sake. We don't always need to be pushed or asked. Sometimes we just love trying to achieve.

STEPS YOU CAN TAKE

STEP 1 – BUILD YOUR HAPPINESS

Look for those moments that produce meaning, engagement, improve relationships, help you to achieve and make you smile. Then build more of them into your daily life. In doing so, you will be truly happy.

- **Positive Emotion.** Look to build your positive emotions about the past, by cultivating gratitude and forgiveness; about the present, by savouring physical pleasures and mindfulness; and about the future, by building hope and optimism.

- **Engagement.** Try to cultivate flow through playing a musical instrument, reading a book, writing, building furniture, fixing a bike, gardening, sports training or performance.

- **Relationships.** Develop strong relationships. The experiences that contribute to well-being, such as great joy, meaning, laughter, a feeling of belonging, and pride in accomplishment are amplified through relationships.

- **Meaning.** This can be derived from belonging to and serving something bigger than the self. For example, connect with religion, family, science, politics, work, justice, the community, or social causes.

- **Accomplishment.** People pursue achievement, competence, success and mastery for its own sake, in a variety of domains, including the workplace, sports, games and hobbies.

STEP 2 – LEARN FROM THE STOICS

Remember that you could die tomorrow, so if you are going to do something, do it now. The Stoics call this *Memento Mori*.

Start living your life by the Stoic virtues of:

- Courage – to do what you want to do
- Wisdom – never stop learning
- Judgement – don't judge others harshly
- Temperance – do things in moderation, apart from drinking of course! Stay sober and appreciate the simple things in life. These are the true key to happiness.

STEP 3 – BE LUCKY

Work at it. Remember that things aren't just given to you. They only happen if you work hard at them. When you work hard, opportunities will arise. Just make sure you take them.

STEP 4 – REMEMBER THE WORLD IS YOUR OYSTER

Everything is open to you if you persist. Keep searching for oysters and remember that all can be opened if you try hard enough. If you persist, you might find a pearl.

STEP 5 – BELIEVE ANYTHING IS POSSIBLE

Make 'Anything Is Possible' your new belief. You can do anything you want to. Remember three little words with a very powerful meaning – YES YOU CAN.

KEY LEARNINGS

- The alcohol-free journey has taken me to a place I had never been to before and I love everything about it. It has led me to my first pearl and I know there are more out there just waiting to be found.

- Everyone views the world in their own unique way, based on their values and beliefs – this is their unique map of life. No two maps are the same.

- Your map is not the territory; it is just the way you view the world. You can change it by changing your beliefs.

- The future has not yet been written. Life is full of opportunities to find the treasures you seek.

- *Memento Mori.* Do it now, do it right now.

- Don't regret anything. Don't become an 'I coulda, I shoulda, I woulda' person.

- Be happy. Look for those moments that produce meaning, engagement, improve relationships, help you to achieve and make you smile. Then build more of them into your daily life. In doing so, you will be truly happy.

- Make 'Anything Is Possible' your new belief.

- YES YOU CAN.

FINAL WORD

I started this book with the Buddhist teaching, *'Under the floor of some poor man's house lies a treasure. But because he does not know of its existence, he does not think he is rich. Similarly, inside one's mind lies truth itself, firm and unfading. Yet because beings see it not, they experience a constant stream of misery. The treasure of truth lies within the house of the mind.'*

You've just got to know where to look.

The search of 'what to look for' and 'where to look for it' became my journey. A journey of discovery and enlightenment. I realised I was looking for happiness. Happiness was not an outcome, or a destination, it was in fact the journey itself, or the way I live my life.

Through following my purpose, living in the present moment, having an optimistic view, and developing strong open relationships with people I love, I found what I was looking for.

And where did I find it? It was both inside me and all around me. Just sitting there waiting to be found. I just needed to make the connection and let it flow through me.

Finding happiness in the way I live my life IS the secret to alcohol-free living and well-being.

Happiness is truly just a mindset. It resides all around us and inside all of us. You just have to let it in.

To find out more about Walking Back To Happiness and stay in touch, go to www.9kmby9am.com and subscribe to our newsletter.

APPENDIX

ALCOHOLOMETER

WALKING BACK TO HAPPINESS
THE SECRET TO ALCOHOL-FREE LIVING & WELL-BEING

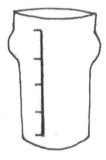
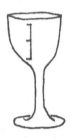
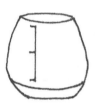

THE DEFINITIVE GUIDE TO HOW MUCH NEAT OR PURE ALCOHOL YOU DRINK

WWW.9KMBY9AM.COM/BOOK

THE DEFINITIVE GUIDE TO HOW MUCH PURE ALCOHOL YOU DRINK?

STEP 1 - Select your drink type and its Alcohol By Volume (ABV).
STEP 2 - Cross reference with the amount you drink. The number in the table is the amount of neat alcohol expressed in litres.
For bespoke amounts multiply the number of pints or bottles by the number in the table.
For example:
50 pints of Beer at 6% ABV is 1.704 litres of neat alcohol.
50 bottles of wine at 13% ABV is 4.875 litres of neat alcohol.
50 bottles of whisky at 40% ABV is 14 litres of neat alcohol.

Bold numbers relate to the more common ABVs.

BEER / LAGER - PURE ALCOHOL IN LITRES   BASED ON PINTS DRUNK

ABV%	PURE ALCOHOL PER PINT (568ML)	1 PINT	5 PINTS	10 PINTS	50 PINTS	100 PINTS	500 PINTS	1000 PINTS
	LITRES	LITRES	LITRES	LITRES	LITRES	LITRES	LITRES	LITRES
3.0%	0.01704	0.01704	0.0852	0.1704	0.852	1.704	8.520	17.040
3.5%	0.01988	0.01988	0.0994	0.1988	0.994	1.988	9.940	19.880
4.0%	**0.02272**	**0.02272**	**0.1136**	**0.2272**	**1.136**	**2.272**	**11.360**	**22.720**
4.5%	0.02556	0.02556	0.1278	0.2556	1.278	2.556	12.780	25.560
5.0%	**0.0284**	**0.02840**	**0.1420**	**0.2840**	**1.420**	**2.840**	**14.200**	**28.400**
5.5%	0.03124	0.03124	0.1562	0.3124	1.562	3.124	15.620	31.240
6.0%	0.03408	0.03408	0.1704	0.3408	1.704	3.408	17.040	34.080
6.5%	0.03692	0.03692	0.1846	0.3692	1.846	3.692	18.460	36.920
7.0%	0.03976	0.03976	0.1988	0.3976	1.988	3.976	19.880	39.760
7.5%	0.0426	0.04260	0.2130	0.4260	2.130	4.260	21.300	42.600
8.0%	0.04544	0.04544	0.2272	0.4544	2.272	4.544	22.720	45.440

WINE - PURE ALCOHOL IN LITRES   BASED ON BOTTLES DRUNK

ABV%	PURE ALCOHOL PER BOTTLE (750ML)	1 BOTTLE	5 BOTTLES	10 BOTTLES	50 BOTTLES	100 BOTTLES	500 BOTTLES	1000 BOTTLES
	LITRES	LITRES	LITRES	LITRES	LITRES	LITRES	LITRES	LITRES
9.0%	0.068	0.068	0.338	0.675	3.375	6.750	33.750	67.500
9.5%	0.071	0.071	0.356	0.713	3.563	7.125	35.625	71.250
10.0%	0.075	0.075	0.375	0.750	3.750	7.500	37.500	75.000
10.5%	0.079	0.079	0.394	0.788	3.938	7.875	39.375	78.750
11.0%	0.083	0.083	0.413	0.825	4.125	8.250	41.250	82.500
11.5%	0.086	0.086	0.431	0.863	4.313	8.625	43.125	86.250
12.0%	0.090	0.090	0.450	0.900	4.500	9.000	45.000	90.000
12.5%	**0.094**	**0.094**	**0.469**	**0.938**	**4.688**	**9.375**	**46.875**	**93.750**
13.0%	0.098	0.098	0.488	0.975	4.875	9.750	48.750	97.500
13.5%	**0.101**	**0.101**	**0.506**	**1.013**	**5.063**	**10.125**	**50.625**	**101.250**
14.0%	0.105	0.105	0.525	1.050	5.250	10.500	52.500	105.000
14.5%	0.109	0.109	0.544	1.088	5.438	10.875	54.375	108.750
15.0%	0.113	0.113	0.563	1.125	5.625	11.250	56.250	112.500

SPIRITS - PURE ALCOHOL IN LITRES   BASED ON BOTTLES DRUNK

ABV%	PURE ALCOHOL PER BOTTLE (700ML)	1 BOTTLE	5 BOTTLES	10 BOTTLES	50 BOTTLES	100 BOTTLES	500 BOTTLES	1000 BOTTLES
	LITRES	LITRES	LITRES	LITRES	LITRES	LITRES	LITRES	LITRES
20%	0.140	0.140	0.700	1.40	7.00	14.00	70.00	140.00
25%	0.175	0.175	0.875	1.75	8.75	17.50	87.50	175.00
30%	0.210	0.210	1.050	2.10	10.50	21.00	105.00	210.00
35%	0.245	0.245	1.225	2.45	12.25	24.50	122.50	245.00
40%	**0.280**	**0.280**	**1.400**	**2.80**	**14.00**	**28.00**	**140.00**	**280.00**
45%	0.315	0.315	1.575	3.15	15.75	31.50	157.50	315.00

Copyright 2022: Nigel Jones

DAILY DRINKING

STEP 1 – Select your drink type and its Alcohol By Volume (ABV).
STEP 2 – Cross reference with the amount you drink. The number in the table is the amount of neat alcohol expressed in litres.
For example:
A pint of beer per day for 1 Year at 6.0% ABV is 12.4392 litres of neat alcohol.
A bottle of wine a day at 12.5% ABV for 1 Year is 34.219 litres of neat alcohol.
A bottle of spirits a week at 40% ABV for 1 Year is 14.560 litres of neat alcohol.

Bold numbers relate to the more common ABVs.

BEER/LAGER – 1 x PINT PER DAY

ABV%	PURE ALCOHOL PER PINT (568ML)	1 WEEK: 7 DAYS (7 PINTS)	1 MONTH: 30 DAYS (30 PINTS)	1 YEAR: 365 DAYS (365 PINTS)	
	LITRES	LITRES	LITRES	LITRES	
3.0%	0.01704	0.1193	0.5112	6.2196	
3.5%	0.01988	0.1392	0.5964	7.2562	
4.0%	**0.02272**	**0.1590**	**0.6816**	**8.2928**	Average Beer/Lager
4.5%	0.02556	0.1789	0.7668	9.3294	
5.0%	**0.02840**	**0.1988**	**0.8520**	**10.3660**	Average Stronger Beer/Lager
5.5%	0.03124	0.2187	0.9372	11.4026	
6.0%	0.03408	0.2386	1.0224	12.4392	
6.5%	0.03692	0.2584	1.1076	13.4758	
7.0%	0.03976	0.2783	1.1928	14.5124	
7.5%	0.04260	0.2982	1.2780	15.5490	
8.0%	0.04544	0.3181	1.3632	16.5856	

WINE – 1 x BOTTLE PER DAY

ABV%	PURE ALCOHOL PER BOTTLE (750ML)	1 WEEK: 7 DAYS (7 BOTTLES)	1 MONTH: 30 DAYS (30 BOTTLES)	1 YEAR: 365 DAYS (365 BOTTLES)	
	LITRES	LITRES	LITRES	LITRES	
9.0%	0.068	0.051	0.038	24.638	
9.5%	0.071	0.499	2.138	26.006	
10.0%	0.075	0.525	2.250	27.375	
10.5%	0.079	0.551	2.363	28.744	
11.0%	0.083	0.578	2.475	30.113	
11.5%	0.086	0.604	2.588	31.481	
12.0%	0.090	0.630	2.700	32.850	
12.5%	**0.094**	**0.656**	**2.813**	**34.219**	Average Bottle White Wine
13.0%	0.098	0.683	2.925	35.588	
13.5%	**0.101**	**0.709**	**3.038**	**36.956**	Average Bottle Red Wine
14.0%	0.105	0.735	3.150	38.325	
14.5%	0.109	0.761	3.263	39.694	
15.0%	0.113	0.788	3.375	41.063	

SPIRITS – 1 x BOTTLE PER WEEK

ABV%	PURE ALCOHOL PER BOTTLE (700ML)	1 WEEK: 7 DAYS (1 BOTTLE)	1 MONTH: 30 DAYS (4.5 BOTTLES)	I YEAR: 52 WEEKS (52 BOTTLES)	
	LITRES	LITRES	LITRES	LITRES	
20%	0.140	0.140	0.630	7.280	
25%	0.175	0.175	0.788	9.100	
30%	0.210	0.210	0.945	10.920	
35%	0.245	0.245	1.103	12.740	
40%	**0.280**	**0.280**	**1.260**	**14.560**	Average Bottle Gin or Whisky
45%	0.315	0.315	1.418	16.380	

Copyright: Nigel Jones

SOURCES

CHAPTER 2

https://www.argumentninja.com/

Alcohol Change UK

Global Burden of Diseases, University of Washington

CHAPTER 3

Charles Duhigg, *The Power of Habit: Why We Do What We Do and How To Change* 2013

https://www.healthline.com/health/mental-health/habit-loop

http://examinedexistence.com/the-habit-loop-the-concept-that-explains-how-habits-form/

https://www.recoveryconnection.com/cycle-addiction/

CHAPTER 4

https://www.recoveryconnection.com/

CHAPTER 5

Source According to Dr. Mohammed Saeed, MD. https://www.intoactionrecovery.com/how-dopamine-drives-our-behavior/

Alcohol Change UK is the operating name of Alcohol Research UK, registered charity no. 1140287, a limited company registered in England and Wales. https://alcoholchange.org.uk/alcohol-facts/fact-sheets/alcohol-statistics

'Dopamine modulates the reward experiences elicited by music' by Laura Ferreri, an associate professor in cognitive psychology at Lyon University.

CHAPTER 7

Amitava Dasgupta, *Critical Issues in Alcohol and Drugs of Abuse Testing (Second Edition)*, 2019

www.drinkaware.co.uk

CHAPTER 8

James Clear, *Atomic Habits* 2018

Chris McHesney, Sean Covey and Jim Huling, *The 4 Disciplines Of Execution* 2021,.

Chris Wilson https://simplifyyourwhy.com/

The Tim Ferris Show #514, interview with *Lululemon* founder Chip Wilson on the art of setting goals https://tim. blog/2021/05/21/chip-wilson-transcript/

One Year No Beer

CHAPTER 9

One Year No Beer

Andy Ramage

Henry David Theroux

Anthony Robbins

CHAPTER 10

One Year No Beer

Andy Ramage

Henry David Theroux

Anthony Robbins

CHAPTER 11

One Year No Beer

Pema Chödrön. In *When Things Fall Apart: Heart Advice for Difficult Times* https://www.themarginalian.org/2017/07/17/when-things-fall-apart-pema-chodron/

Abraham Maslow, *A Theory of Human Motivation* 2013

Mary Oliver, *The Summer Day*

Rich Roll Episode 633 with Rainn Wilson and Reza Aslan
https://www.richroll.com/podcast/rainn-reza-633/

CHAPTER 12

Rabbi Mordecai Finley - https://www.rabbifinley.com/

Anthony Robbins - https://www.tonyrobbins.com/stories/unleash-the-power/change-your-story/

Dan Siegel - https://drdansiegel.com/hand-model-of-the-brain/

Henry David Thoreau, *Walden* 2018

Dan Harris, *10% Happier* 2017

Annie Grace, *Naked Mind* 2018

Craig Beck, *Alcohol Lied to Me*

Victor Frankl, *Man's Search for Meaning* 2004

Anthony Robbins, *Awaken the Giant Within* 2001

The Daily Stoic - https://dailystoic.com/

The 5AM Miracle Podcast - https://www.jeffsanders.com/podcast/

Rich Roll - https://www.richroll.com/

Tara Brach - https://www.tarabrach.com/

CHAPTER 13

Gary Keller, *The One Thing* 2014

Kelly McGonigal, *The Willpower Instinct* 2013

Roy F. Baumeister, *Willpower: Why Self-control is the Secret to Success* 2012

One Year No Beer

Dan Millman

Catarina Lino *www.positivepsychology.com*

Baba Shiv

CHAPTER 15

Tara Brach & Jack Kornfield Podcast

Holly J. Bertone, CNHP, PMP and Crystal Hoshaw - https://www.healthline.com/health/mental-health/types-of-meditation#takeaway

Chopra - https://chopra.com/articles/how-to-be-mindful-without-meditation

Mind Body Green - https://www.mindbodygreen.com/articles/the-12-major-types-of-meditation-explained-simply

Eckhart Tolle, *The Power of Now* 2001

Dan Siegel, *Aware*

Dan Harris, *10% Happier* 2017

Pedram Shojai, *The Urban Monk* 2017

CHAPTER 16

Ryan Holiday, *Stillness Is The Key* 2020

Psychology Today - https://www.psychologytoday.com/us/basics/gratitude

Orion Philosophy - https://www.orionphilosophy.com/stoic-blog/stoic-quotes-on-discipline

Daily Stoic - https://dailystoic.com/gratitude/

Rick Hanson https://www.rickhanson.net/gratitude-2/

Tara Brach Podcast - Gratitude (25th November 2021)

Rich Roll Podcast - Raghunath Cappo (Episode 583)

Anthony Robbins

CHAPTER 17

John Seabrook - https://www.newyorker.com/magazine/2021/09/27/an-ex-drinkers-search-for-a-sober-buzz

Drinkaware - https://www.drinkaware.co.uk/facts/alcoholic-drinks-and-units/difference-between-alcoholic-and-non-alcoholic-beers

CHAPTER 18

Gary Keller, *The One Thing* 2014

Arianna Huffington, *The Sleep Revolution, Transforming Your Life One Night At A Time* 2017

http://theshawnstevensonmodel.com/podcasts/

https://www.oneyearnobeer.com/maximize-your-potential-through-better-sleep-health/

https://www.everydayhealth.com/sleep/insomnia/resetting-your-clock.aspx

Rafael Pelayo, MD, Clinical Professor at the Stanford Sleep Disorders Clinic, and Stanford University School of Medicine, California.

CHAPTER 19

Conqueror virtual walk app

Forest Bathing: How Trees Can Help You Find Health and Happiness 2018 by Dr. Qing Li

CHAPTER 20

DRINKAWARE

NHS

CHAPTER 21

The Daily Stoic Podcast https://www.dailystoic.com

Tara Brach Podcast https://www.tarabrach.com/

BBC Bitesize https://www.bbc.co.uk/bitesize/

Wabi Sabi https://en.wikipedia.org/wiki/Wabi-sabi

Alan Watts, *The Way of Zen* 1999

The Dalai Lama, *The Wheel of Life – Buddhist Perspectives on Cause and Effect* 2016

Jonathan Landaw, Stephan Bodian, Gurrun Buhnemann, *Buddhism For Dummies, Second Edition* 2019

Maitreya Buddha text adapted from a translation by Glen Mullin

Beth Kempton, *Wabi Sabi: Japanese Wisdom for a Perfectly Imperfect Life* 2018

Ryan Holiday, *Ego is the Enemy* 2017

Tara Talks: The Wisdom of Impermanence, January 2022 https://www.youtube.com/watch?v=Y8nw-CS1cRU

CHAPTER 23
One Year No Beer

CHAPTER 27

Arthur C. Brooks, *From Strength to Strength: Finding Success, Happiness and Deep Purpose in the Second Half of Life* 2022

Bronnie Ware, *The Top Five Regrets of the Dying* 2019

Martin Seligman – the PERMA Theory of Wellbeing

Positive Psychology Centre https://ppc.sas.upenn.edu/learn-more/perma-theory-well-being-and-perma-workshops

Matthew McConaughey Oscars Acceptance 2014 https://genius.com/Matthew-mcconaughey-bes...

Printed in Great Britain
by Amazon

21760741R00148